The Mission of the National Aphasi[a] understanding of aphasia and provi[...] caregivers.

The NAA envisions a society in which aphasia is a commonly understood word and where all persons with aphasia, regardless of individual differences, their families, health professionals, and the public have access to appropriate education and resources that would enhance their potential for an acceptable quality of life.

Board of Directors

Darlene S. Williamson, M.S., CCC-SLP, President

Daniel Martin, Treasurer

Barbara Kessler, Vice President Community Outreach & Education

Thomas G. Broussard Jr. Ph.D, Vice President Community Outreach & Education

Members

Elaine Adler

Carol Kirshner, Secretary

Howard S. Kirshner, M.D., Vice President Research & Medical Issues

Peter Turkeltaub, M.D., Ph.D., Vice President Research & Medical Issues

Steve Kessler, Vice President Strategic Planning

Chad Ruble, Vice President Innovation & Programming

Author: Melissa Ford

Editor: Randall Klein

Copyright © 2020 National Aphasia Association

All rights reserved

CONTENTS

Welcome	5
Introduction	6
Chapter 1: Caregiver Facts and Figures	10
Chapter 2: A Crash Course in Aphasia	13
Chapter 3: Navigating a New Normal	18
Chapter 4: Getting Organized	21
Chapter 5: Becoming an Advocate	26
Chapter 6: How to Be a Good Question Asker (and Answer Keeper)	29
Chapter 7: Communication Tips and Tools	32
Chapter 8: Explaining Aphasia to Other People	37
Chapter 9: Financial Realities of Aphasia	42
Chapter 10: Finding Calm on the Stormy Seas	46
Chapter 11: Finding Your Circles of Support	49
Chapter 12: You've Delegated… Now What?	55
Chapter 13: Care for the Caregiver	60
Chapter 14: Dealing with Your Feelings	66
Chapter 15: Finding Care for the Caregiver	71
Thank You	76
Appendix I	77
Appendix II	78

WELCOME

It is with great pleasure that the National Aphasia Association makes this book on caregiving available to the aphasia community. It is our mission to serve families living with aphasia, with an emphasis on the word *family*. We know that aphasia affects the whole family, indeed, the person's whole sphere of influence. When an individual experiences a stroke or other brain trauma that leads to aphasia, life changes in an instant.

We recognize that the road to a future with aphasia can be a rocky one, with many twists and turns. Aphasia is a life-long condition. No one is prepared for all the adaptations that will need to be made. It is our intent that this book will provide some help navigating the path which leads to a "new normal."

This document was prepared by the NAA team and reviewed by caregivers who gave us their expert input. Not all the information will apply to every family and not every family will be in a position to use all of the suggestions. Take from it what you find most helpful and what makes the most sense for your situation.

Most importantly, this should be a dynamic book. We've compiled our thoughts, but you'll see in the final chapter that we welcome *your* thoughts. Please use the linked form in the final chapter to give us your helpful hints and suggestions. If you share what worked best for you, we can include the information in the next version to provide a much more comprehensive guide for all caregivers.

The NAA has a proud history of service to the aphasia community. We hope you enjoy this latest initiative, we hope you share the information, and we hope you continue to engage with and support the NAA.

Darlene S. Williamson
President, National Aphasia Association

INTRODUCTION

If you're holding this book, it means someone you love has aphasia.

It may be a husband or wife. A sibling, parent, or child. It may even be a friend. Their life has changed, and now your life is changing, too. You've entered the realm of caregiver, and that can be a very disorienting place to find your footing.

Luckily, you have this guide to help you along. Together, we're going to go through advice that might make your journey a little easier. We can't promise that it will all go smoothly, but when bumps rise up in the road, we'll be alongside you to help you step over them. Let's first figure out where you are and how to best use this book.

What Is a Caregiver?

This book is for *all* caregivers, from primary caregivers involved in the day-to-day life of the person with aphasia to faraway caregivers who are providing aid from other locations.

We are defining a caregiver as **any individual who is voluntarily helping a person with aphasia navigate this communication disorder**. That care may be physical, emotional, or financial in nature.

So we'll start with a thank you. You may not hear it often enough, but you play a necessary part in someone else's life. Thank you for providing support and being the type of person on which other people can rely.

What Will You Find in This Book?

Once you leave the introduction, the book is divided into three main sections. In the first section, you'll find your footing. You'll learn important facts about caregiving and aphasia.

In the second section, you'll be given valuable, concrete tips for getting yourself organized, learning how to be an advocate, and talking about the financial side of aphasia. While some of the advice covers that time period at the beginning of an aphasia journey, where the person may still be in the hospital or newly diagnosed, other ideas can be implemented at any point.

In the final section, we'll talk about gathering support, navigating relationships, and taking care of yourself, including processing the complex feelings that arise when you're a caregiver for someone with aphasia.

How to Use This Book

This book is, first and foremost, a source of comfort reminding you that you're not alone. In fact, the National Aphasia Association is an email away.

It's also a resource for information, helping you think through the questions to ask, the facts to keep at the ready, and the options out there. While you're helping the person with aphasia, we want to help you feel energized and organized. Think of this book like the oxygen mask that you're supposed to secure before helping others in an emergency. You matter, too, and we want to make sure that you have the support you need in order to do your important job.

You don't need to read this book from cover to cover. This book reviews the basic forms of aphasia––from the sudden onset of Broca's aphasia that can happen after a stroke, to the slow loss of words that comes with primary progressive aphasia. You may be at the hospital, or you may be at home. You may be at the very start of an aphasia journey, eager for any and all information, or you may be several years into caregiving and looking for additional advice to make day-to-day life a little easier. As we said, this book is for all caregivers, which means that sometimes you'll encounter paragraphs or even chapters that don't apply to your situation.

In those cases, skip over the words. Your time is precious. Those chapters will always be there if your information needs change.

Lastly, this book is a place to record information. You are going to receive a lot of information, and you need a place to keep it. We've provided worksheets and empty spaces so you can keep advice and answers in one place. So feel free to write in this book––we hope you do.

Being a Successful Caregiver

This book will help you to be a successful caregiver. Being a caregiver means being there for another person without losing yourself in the process. We know––easier said than done, but the way forward is encapsulated in a 2000-year-old idea from the philosopher Hillel.

This very smart person asked three vital questions that apply to caregiving:

    1. If I am not for myself, who will be for me?

    2. If I am only for myself, what am I?

    3. And if now now, when?

If you're not taking care of yourself in the process, who is taking care of you? Even if you have your own caregiving team (and we will help you assemble a small one in a future chapter), you need to remember yourself in this caregiving equation. Get sleep, eat food, and make sure your own needs are being met.

However, if you're not putting the person in need front and center, you're not caregiving. It can be very difficult to have your day-to-day life become about someone else. This book is about understanding how to best be there for another person.

Lastly, whenever caregiving gets overwhelming, it can be helpful to remember that what is happening today will not be happening forever. Tomorrow may be better or worse; the only thing definite is that it will be different. Therefore, balance your needs and the other person's needs to create an equation that adds up to good health and peace of heart for all.

Secure Your Own Mask

Keeping with that oxygen mask analogy, it's very important that your needs get attention, too. You can't support others when you're struggling yourself. Take to heart the words from Jo Horne's "Caregiver Bill of Rights." It begins with this truism: "I have the right to take care of myself. This is not an act of selfishness. It will give me the ability to take better care of my loved one."

A quick Google search will bring you to the rest of your rights. Say the statements aloud (yes, even if it feels a little silly to speak to yourself) to remind yourself to pay attention to your own endurance and emotions.

Congratulations—you're now ready to dive into caregiving without losing yourself in the process. You know how to treat yourself and expect to be treated.

You Can Do This

It's time to dive into the nuts and bolts of supporting a person with aphasia. But before you do, let me tell you a secret: You can do this. Okay, that wasn't really a secret, but it's an important reminder to tuck into the back of your head and say to yourself whenever your day gets overwhelming. You can do this.

Before you think something unhelpful like, "...but I can't do this!" let us remind you that you already know how to be a good caregiver from other areas of your life. We're willing to bet that you already have a lot of experience with tenacity, patience, and empathy. And that is what a caregiver does. A caregiver is someone who creates a safe way forward through a situation, something you have probably done many times in your life before aphasia knocked on your door.

For instance, one way to create that safe way forward is to comfort those around you, namely the person (or people) at the center of the crisis. True caregivers are the people who know it's a marathon, not a sprint, which means they stick around after the initial shock wears off, still providing comfort and support. Think back to other times you've offered comfort to another person, and use that memory as a reminder that you have what it takes to be an effective caregiver. You just need to apply what you know from other facets of your life.

Anytime you doubt yourself, anytime you need a pick-me-up, anytime you need someone to hold you up for a moment so you can take a deep breath and return to doing your important work, turn to this page and look at these words:

You can do this.

Remember that, and let's get started.

CHAPTER 1: CAREGIVER FACTS AND FIGURES

Being thrust into the role of caregiver and leaving behind your pre-aphasia life can be a lonely experience, but rest assured, you are not alone. According to the National Family Caregivers Association, there are around 65 million caregivers in the United States right now. Compare that to the total population of adults in the last census (234.5 million) and almost a third of the people around you are caregivers.

Okay... so where are they hiding? Let's start with caregiver organizations and then speak specifically about aphasia support.

Caregiver Organizations

We've rounded up a list of caregiving organizations. The NAA does not officially endorse any of these organizations, but all are potentially useful resources.

Caregiver Action Network (caregiveraction.org)

"Caregiver Action Network is the nation's leading family caregiver organization working to improve the quality of life for the more than 90 million Americans who care for loved ones with chronic conditions, disabilities, disease, or the frailties of old age."

Caregiver Support Services (caregiversupportservices.com)

"Caregiver Support Services (CSS) is a non-profit organization with a 501(c) (3) tax-exempt status. CSS was founded in 1997 by Terrence and Eboni Green, a husband and wife team, after the couple recognized that most individuals who provide care for a loved one or client do not know where to start when it comes to gathering and coordinating resources and services."

Caring.com (caring.com)

"In 2007, a few friends who were each caring for an aging parent noticed a lack of information online to help them navigate the complexities of caregiving. Not finding the one-stop online resource they needed, they decided to create it themselves. The result was Caring.com."

Family Caregiver Alliance (caregiver.org/pilotIntegration/indexPersistent.html?uri=%2F)

"Founded in the late 1970s, Family Caregiver Alliance is the first community-based non-profit organization in the country to address the needs of families and friends providing long-term care for loved ones at home. FCA, as a public voice for caregivers, shines light on the challenges caregivers face daily and champions their cause through education, services, and advocacy. The services, education programs, and resources FCA provides are designed with caregivers' needs in mind and offer support, tailored information, and tools to manage the complex demands of caregiving."

Lotsa Helping Hands (lotsahelpinghands.com)

"Lotsa Helping Hands powers online caring communities that help restore health and balance to caregivers' lives. Our service brings together caregivers and volunteers through online communities that organize daily life during times of medical crisis or caregiver exhaustion in neighborhoods and communities worldwide. Caregivers benefit from the gifts of much-needed help, emotional support, and peace of mind, while volunteers find meaning in giving back to those in need."

National Alliance for Caregiving (caregiving.org)

"Established in 1996, the National Alliance for Caregiving is a non-profit coalition of national organizations focusing on advancing family caregiving through research, innovation, and advocacy. The Alliance conducts research, does policy analysis, develops national best-practice programs, and works to increase public awareness of family caregiving issues."

Well Spouse Association (wellspouse.org)

"The Well Spouse Association, a nonprofit 501(c)(3) membership organization, advocates for and addresses the needs of individuals caring for a chronically ill and/or disabled spouse/partner. We offer peer-to-peer support and educate health care professionals and the general public about the special challenges and unique issues "well" spouses face every day."

Gathering Aphasia Support

All of the above resources can provide general caregiver support. But it's also important to connect with other people who are specifically helping another person navigate aphasia. If your loved one is still in the hospital, turn to the National Aphasia Association's site (aphasia.org) for caregiver resources or the NAA's Facebook page (facebook.com/NatlAphasiaAssoc/) for conversation with other caregivers.

Once you're in treatment, seek out a caregiver support group within your speech clinic or your neurology group. If you're having trouble locating an aphasia support group aimed at caregivers, enter your ZIP Code into our database (aphasia.org/site/) and reach out to clinics within your area to see if they already have an established group or would be open to starting one if enough interest exists.

At the end of the day, you're far from alone, but you will need to reach out to others in order to find caregiver support. Believe us, it's worth the effort because you'll find a group of people who understand what you're going through and are happy to pool together advice and share ideas that can make your journey a little bit easier.

Now that you know how to find others to walk with you on this journey, let's get the lay of the land and figure out the basics of aphasia—from the different types, to how your life changes when you have aphasia.

CHAPTER 2: A CRASH COURSE IN APHASIA

In 2016, the NAA conducted a survey to discover how much the general public knew about aphasia. Only 8.8% of respondents knew what aphasia was and correctly identified it as a language disorder. That means that the other 91.2% have no clue what you're talking about when you first tell them that your loved one has aphasia.

Maybe you were in that 91.2% before aphasia entered your life. But now that it's all around you, you've gotten a crash course in aphasia. If you've been living in this world for a while, feel free to skip this chapter. But if you're just getting your bearings, dive in, and we'll give you the lay of the land.

Types of Aphasia

We don't want to go too deeply into the various types of aphasia, but we want to give you a base of understanding so you can follow conversations with doctors or speech therapists, ask relevant questions, and conduct your own research on your particular form of aphasia. So use this as a jumping-off point to understand how aphasia differs from person to person, and use it to find additional details about this communication disorder. Every person with aphasia is unique, therefore every person's aphasia presents uniquely from every other person's aphasia. We are providing guidelines that will help you to generally recognize what your loved one is experiencing. Remember, aphasia is a difficulty using language. It is not an intellectual deficit, it is not psychiatric, and it is not motor or muscle-based.

Aphasia types look at a number of factors:
- Does speech come easily (even if it doesn't always make sense) and words are flowing without effort?
- Does the person understand spoken language; can they follow what is being said to them?
- Can the person repeat a phrase back to you?

In some forms of aphasia, the words will flow easily, but they won't make any sense. In other forms of aphasia, the words will be difficult to produce, but you may be able to understand what is trying to be said. There are basically as many presentations of aphasia as there are people with aphasia because each and every person is unique, although their language does fall into categories.

Global

This is the most severe form of aphasia. It significantly alters all four of the language components: comprehension, reading, writing, and speaking. The person can't speak easily, nor can they repeat a word back to you. They don't understand spoken language. Global aphasia may be a temporary state, such as immediately following a stroke, that improves over time. But in some cases of severe brain damage, the situation may be permanent. Even if global aphasia persists, there are ways to support communication and live successfully.

Broca's Aphasia

Words don't come easily, and when they do, it's only a word or short phrases at a time. They may understand everything being said to them, but they can't respond. Their vocabulary is affected, and they lose access to calling up and using even familiar words. This is a form of "non-fluent" aphasia, and it's called that because speech comes out haltingly.

Wernicke's Aphasia

Words flow very easily, but they typically don't make sense when strung together in sentences. People with Wernicke's aphasia may not be able to understand what is being said to them. Their own speech may be peppered with irrelevant or nonsense words, though they may hear their speech as normal and not comprehend why other people can't understand them. This is a form of "fluent" aphasia because the words flow out of the mouth easily.

Anomic Aphasia

Speech is filled with circumlocutions -- talking around the thing they want to talk about because they're missing a word -- and expressions of frustration. While the person may understand spoken conversations and directions, and even be able to read adequately, they struggle with writing or finding the nouns and verbs they want with spoken speech.

Primary Progressive Aphasia

This is the only form of aphasia that gets worse over time. While other forms of aphasia come on suddenly due to a head injury or stroke and then either remain the same or improve over time, this form of aphasia comes on slowly and worsens over months or years. Primary progressive aphasia is a neurological syndrome caused by brain tissue deteriorating. There is currently no cure for primary progressive aphasia, but there are ways to help maintain communication ability longer.

Your Aphasia Questions

You are probably filled with questions if you're encountering aphasia for the first time and trying to get your bearings. We've tried to answer some of them below, and while our list won't contain everything churning in your mind, we will at least give you a starting point for understanding the diagnosis. We'll go deeper into these questions in the next section.

Can you tell me the basics of aphasia?

It's an acquired communication disorder, which means that it's something that happens during the course of life instead of being present from birth. It affects the person's ability to process language but does not affect intelligence. While it is more common in older people, it can be acquired following a stroke or brain trauma at any age.

What causes aphasia?

The most common cause of aphasia is a stroke. In fact, about 25% - 40% of stroke survivors acquire aphasia. Other causes include traumatic brain injury or a brain tumor. Additionally, with primary progressive aphasia (see above), there is a neurological cause.

Does it always look the same?

Aphasia presents differently depending on the type (see above) or severity. In a mild form, you may not be able to tell the person is having difficulty forming words. In other cases, it is immediately apparent that the person is having trouble using language. It affects speech, understanding, writing, and reading differently.

Do many people have aphasia?

Yes -- which is why it was so surprising to discover that only 8.8% of the general public knows about aphasia. It affects two million Americans, and it's more common than other well-known conditions such as Parkinson's disease, cerebral palsy, or muscular dystrophy.

Are there any other problems that accompany aphasia?

Damage to the left side of the brain (where a lot of language processing is done) affects the right side of the body, so when a person has aphasia, they may also have weakness or paralysis in their right arm and/or leg.

It is important to note that there are two other conditions that can occur alongside aphasia.

The first is apraxia. Apraxia of speech is a condition where the person has lost the ability to voluntarily make the movements necessary for speech, without any paralysis or weakness in the muscles. Apraxia can also occur in the arms or hands, making it difficult for the person to gesture. It is especially frustrating for the individual because they can conceptualize what they want to say or do with arms, but the connection to make the movement has been affected. Apraxia can often be confused with Broca's type aphasia; your speech therapist will make this diagnosis and provide treatment. Treatment for apraxia is often long and arduous.

The second is dysarthria. Dysarthria is a weakness in the oral muscles (lips, tongue, cheeks) that causes speech to be slow and slurred, and therefore can be difficult to understand. These same muscles are responsible for swallowing. Again, your speech therapist will be able to identify dysarthria and prepare treatment that will help restore the use of the muscles.

How long will it take for the person to recover?

In the case of primary progressive aphasia, speech difficulties will get progressively worse, not better. In the case of aphasia after a stroke or head injury, improvement can take weeks, months, or years. It's also important to remember that "complete recovery" isn't the only possibility. Speech can improve year after year, decade after decade, especially with speech therapy. Living successfully with aphasia may be the best outcome.

How is aphasia treated?

Aphasia is usually treated by a speech-language pathologist who will work to recover speech and language, as well as support new communication methods and strategies that work for the individual and the family.

Is intelligence affected?

No -- as mentioned above, people with aphasia may have difficulty producing words, but their intelligence is intact. Their ideas, thoughts, and knowledge are still in their head -- it's just communicating those ideas, thoughts, and knowledge that is interrupted.

Does that mean the person with aphasia can return to their job or old life?

Maybe. If speech and language are central to a person's job, it may make work difficult. Activities that require a lot of speaking, reading, and writing may be difficult temporarily or indefinitely. Because every case of aphasia is different, it's impossible to predict how one person's aphasia will change the course of their life.

At this point, you may have more questions than answers. Let's dive deeper into navigating this new normal in the final chapter of section one before we move into our focus on caregiving and care*givers*. Like you.

CHAPTER 3: NAVIGATING A NEW NORMAL

Aphasia has seeped into every aspect of your day-to-day world. You know the basic types of aphasia and why it occurs, but now it's time to look at the way your life may change due to aphasia. Is aphasia difficult? Of course. It is a very stressful condition, but people also report hope, finding joy in moments they may have missed before aphasia, as well as closer relationships. While aphasia may feel like it has more "bad" aspects than good ones, there are moments of light once you acclimate yourself to the new normal.

What Will Change?

The glib answer is "everything," but take a step back. Your loved one is still your loved one. They still have the same intelligence and character traits you know and love. They are themselves, albeit with a reduced capacity to communicate.

A 2018 study out of the Cleveland Clinic looked at 1,195 people after a stroke to measure the psychological effects and hidden quality-of-life impacts of the condition. More than half voiced frustration with social and work-related activities. What powered their life prior to the stroke -- social interactions and meaningful work -- now often requires greater effort. And while this may seem obvious, it actually serves as an important reminder: adjust your expectations.

Expectations

Expectations are both a blessing and a curse when it comes to aphasia. On one hand, you need to have expectations. Why else would you invest time in speech therapy if you didn't *expect* it would help your loved one communicate better? On the other hand, your expectations may cause frustration because every aphasia situation is different. What works easily for one person may not work for your loved one, or vice versa.

Things may go slower than you wish, especially when it comes to recovery. Actually, scratch that: things *will* go slower than you wish because even one minute being unable to communicate feels too long. Moreover, recovery may look different from what exists in your head when you first hear the word "aphasia."

It may help to mentally pack all your expectations in a virtual suitcase, much as you bring various items from home with you on a trip. Sometimes these expectations are helpful, making you feel more settled in an unfamiliar situation. But sometimes these expectations need to be left behind in your mental hotel room so you can explore the reality of the space around you. When you're feeling overwhelmed, ask yourself if your frustration stems from expectations. If they do, try setting them aside for a moment to look at the situation from a new angle.

Everyone Is Different

Every person is different, so it follows that every aphasia recovery is different. Some people will regain their speech after a stroke. Some people will not. Some people will lose their speech slowly with primary progressive aphasia. Some people will lose their speech quickly. There is no "normal" when it comes to aphasia.

And it may take you time to grow comfortable with your new normal. It is helpful to know that you will find your footing. There will be moments of equilibrium, but those will shift, along with your situation and the recovery process for the person you are caring for.

It may help to pause for a second in reading this booklet and set a new goal. Instead of focusing on recovery -- whatever the term "recovery" means to you -- ask yourself how you can take your new normal and make it incrementally better. Instead of thinking about the way things were before aphasia entered your life, look at life now, and ask yourself what could change by the end of the day to take you one step closer to things being better in the evening than they were in the morning. The situation becomes more manageable when you think about the tiny steps forward rather than the giant leaps before you.

Thrust into Caregiving

So that's how your loved one's life will change. And that is partially how your life will change, too. But your life is now about aphasia AND caregiving, and that is the weight we'll address for the rest of this booklet.

Being a caregiver isn't something we really choose. It's a role we're thrust into when life changes for a loved one and we need to step in and help. Adults like being autonomous, so this role may come with a lot of frustration because it was (1) chosen for you and (2) it's not always enjoyable. Who wants to see their loved one frustrated or hurt?

Moreover, this position comes without any guidance. Unlike your job, which likely came with knowledge imparted by a degree or a training program, you are expected to jump into caregiving without the benefit of an on-ramp. It can be difficult to get your bearings.

The short answer is there is no "right" or "wrong" when it comes to caregiving, and no single way to do things.

But the most important point is that YOUR emotions need addressing, too. It's not just your loved one who has had their life turned upside down. Your life has changed as well, and that is no small thing.

Going from Doing to Waiting

Sometimes doing nothing will be doing something. So much of this situation will be out of your control, and being a caregiver is often about waiting. Understanding there is nothing you can do to speed along recovery is one of the most difficult but important lessons learned from being a caregiver. If you're accustomed to making things happen, it can be incredibly frustrating to sit still and wait for something to happen, but patience is part of the job.

It may help to remember that you're not actually doing "nothing." You're actually doing something very important every single second of the day: you're holding hope when it's too hard for your loved one to carry it. Being the hoper, the cheerleader, and the energy provider to move things forward may be the most important task of caregiving, and those things can happen whenever you choose to be the hoper, cheerleader, and energy provider.

What about You?

Well, what about you? This book *is* about you and is meant to support you through a difficult time. Can you keep working? Seeing your friends? Engaging in hobbies or going on business trips? In other words, can you keep being you while you're caregiving?

Yes.

The point of caregiving is not to lose everything in your life while you help your loved one. Whatever will help you remain a solid and steady presence in your loved one's life should remain part of your world. That includes working without guilt while you're caregiving because you simultaneously need to earn a paycheck, taking care of your emotional health by recharging so you can be there for your loved one, or seeking therapy to help you adjust to the new normal.

Everyone needs a purpose in life, and it doesn't help your loved one if you cast yours aside. You need something outside the caregiver experience, and that is a lesson we will not allow you to forget as you make your way through this booklet. Let's dive in.

CHAPTER 4: GETTING ORGANIZED

Caregivers have a lot of information thrown their way and the deluge of facts, figures, and appointments never stop for as long as you're in that caregiver role. Your greatest weapon in the fight to keep all those facts, figures, and appointments from slipping through the cracks is a good organizational system that allows you to take that information out of your mind, and to free up your mental space so you can take actual breaks from your caregiver mindset.

Spiral Notebooks Are Your Friends

A simple spiral notebook, purchased from any grocery store or office supply store, is the best receptacle for all the information you'll need to record. You'll use it to create a modified bullet journal, the invention of Ryder Carroll. A bullet journal is a simple way to capture thoughts, facts, and to-do list items in a single space. His amazing system helps you remember everything the doctor says, an app that someone tells you about in the waiting room, or a reminder that you need to contact your loved one's boss to give them an update on the situation.

Get a spiral notebook, and we'll help you set it up. In fact, if you want to take a quick peek at Appendix I, you'll see a preview of what we'll talk about below.

First Type of Page: Calendar Spread

Open the notebook to the first page. Write the name of the month at the top. Then number down the left side of the page, one day per line. Write the day of the week as a single letter beside the number. Depending on the size of your
notebook, you will probably need to use a two-page spread, though you may only use a few lines on the second page.

For example:

September 2019

1 S
2 M

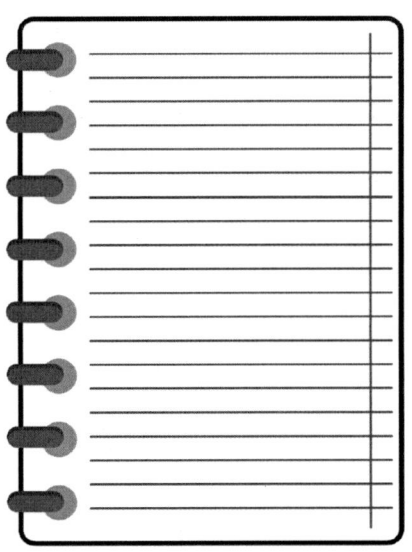

3 T
4 W

At the end of each day, you will write one sentence about the day. It may be an accomplishment you want to remember or a setback you need to track. It can be difficult to see the scope of improvement if you don't pause to record those moments that define the day. A sample notebook page may look like this:

September 2019

1 S Jane came to visit, but Jim couldn't remember her name.
2 M Speech therapy in the morning. Jim does better when we do therapy earlier.
3 T Jim started using thumbs up or thumbs down for yes or no. Big improvement!
4 W Jim was too tired for speech therapy. He's frustrated.
5 T Jane came again. Jim called her Jane and she cried with relief. (I did, too.)
6 F Allison canceled speech therapy. Went to park and used flowers to name colors.
7 S Jim made very funny joke about mixing up bats and hats.

Looking back on the notes, it's easy to see the ups and downs of an average week. This type of record-keeping will become invaluable, jogging your memory so you can see progress. They are pages you can return to when you're feeling discouraged to see how far you've come.

Second Type of Page: Daily Entries

Flip to the third page in your notebook and write the date on the first line, flush left. Underneath the date, take notes as you go through your day. Any action items––things you need to do––get a square next to them. You'll be able to scan down your page at the end of the day and see any unchecked squares, which will remind you of things you need to get done. In our example, the person needs to remember to bring Jim a pillow.

Any non-action items, things you simply want to remember, get a dot next to them. These are suggestions from the speech therapist, moments you want to remember, apps you want to check out in the future, or ideas that you want to make sure don't slip your mind.

Finally, questions begin with a question mark. Make sure that the question mark stands out so you'll notice your questions whenever you get a chance to ask them.

THE APHASIA CAREGIVER GUIDE

September 1
- ☐ Bring Jim pillow
- ● Allison says that thumbs up or thumbs down gestures can help Jim communicate what he wants.
- ● New words Jim can say right now:
  - Oh no
  - Up (sometimes uses it to mean "yes")
  - Hi
  - You
  - Red
- ❓ Ask Dr. Ambrin about the medication he mentioned yesterday.

Every day, write the new date and start note-taking anew. Don't forget to flip back through the pages, looking for any outstanding action items or unasked questions. Or if you're worried about forgetting to do something, recopy it under the new date. Some days, you may have many notes, and other days, you may have nothing written. The point of this system is to record the things YOU want to remember, not to feel pressured to write when there is nothing to write.

What happens when you get to a new month? The system starts again. Flip the page and begin your new two-page monthly spread so you have a place to sum up the day with a single thought. Then flip the page again and write the first day of the month and start the daily entries. Don't forget to copy over anything undone or unasked from the previous month.

You will be able to keep several months of information––at least six months, maybe more––in a single notebook. Always keep your current caregiver notebook with you so you'll be able to take thoughts out of your brain and put them on the page for safekeeping.

Folders Are Your Friend, Too

You're also going to get many handouts. There will be the worksheets or progress reports for your loved one as well as receipts, prescriptions, or referrals. You will need a simple folder with pockets, once again purchased at any grocery store or office supply store, so you have a single space for placing all of these pieces of paper.

One side of the folder will be incoming paperwork: bills you need to pay, prescriptions you need to fill, or referrals you need to use. The other side of the folder will be archivable paperwork, such as receipts, test results, or fact sheets. This will help you quickly find anything on the left side, or "to do" section of the folder, as well as anything on the right side, or "done" section of the folder.

While a folder isn't the largest thing to carry with you, if you're feeling overwhelmed, consider moving those archivable pieces of paper out of the folder and transferring them to a box or a larger accordion folder in your home so you can quickly find them again. But before you do, turn them into a PDF you can store on your phone.

Any phone with a camera can be turned into a "scanner" with a simple app, such as

Scanner or Scanner Pro. An app uses the camera on your phone to make a copy of the paper that you can keep with you. If you don't want to download a free app, you can also snap a quick picture of the paper and keep that on your camera roll in case you need to access it while you're away from home.

Information to Have at Your Fingertips

Whether you're still in the hospital following your loved one's stroke or traumatic brain injury, or well into the world of aphasia outside the hospital, there are pieces of information you'll want to have at your fingertips. You can use the back pages of your caregiver notebook to copy down these often-used names and numbers in order to have them handy at all times.

- Any medications the person takes and specific instructions for that medication.
- List of any allergies (especially medication or food allergies) any staff needs to know about for treating your loved one.
- The names of any procedures or tests and the dates they were done.
- Name of insurance company, name, and direct phone number of a representative at the company, and your loved one's identification number from the card.
- A backup contact at the insurance company in case your main agent is ever out of town.
- Names and phone numbers for people in the hospital billing department if you're still in the hospital.
- Name and phone number of any case managers or patient advocates at the hospital.
- Name and contact information for all therapists (speech, physical, occupational, etc).

Having all of this information on one page will give you a quick place to turn to when you're seeking an answer, and it will enable you to hand off care of your loved one to someone else in case of an emergency because they will have everything they need to dive in.

Start a Conversation Log

You may also want to start a page to log conversations in the back of your caregiver notebook. This is a place to record phone calls and face-to-face conversations concerning your loved one's care so you can refer back to conversations in the future. What type of information will you want to record? Start with the date, the person you spoke to, and the content of the conversation, including any action items that come out of the call.

For example:

Conversation Log

- 9/1/19: Spoke to Dana at the insurance company. She promised to look into re-

imbursement for August speech therapy session that wasn't covered.
- 9/5/19: Spoke to Dr. Ambrin and he said Jim would qualify for aphasia trial at the hospital. Follow up with him next Wednesday after he has spoken to the team.
- 9/9/19: Spoke to Dana again at insurance company. She said the reimbursement was sent this morning. Contact her again if I don't have it by the end of the week.

Keeping track of any and all conversations pertaining to your loved one's care will help you stay on top of things while not wasting precious headspace remembering them.

Now that you're organized, it's time to talk about being your loved one's advocate. Even if you're old hat in the advocacy game, we hope our tips will give you easy ways to navigate the system, get your loved one the best care possible, and stay calm in the process.

CHAPTER 5: BECOMING AN ADVOCATE

If you're an adult, you are well-versed in being your own advocate. You have a lifetime of experience navigating systems to get what you need and speaking up when you don't. But even well-seasoned advocates will find themselves drained when trying to be an advocate for their loved one during a health crisis. Fortunately, there are people and information out there to help you.

Find Out What You Need

You'll run into roadblocks. It's just a given when you're navigating a new situation. There are rules and regulations that people need to follow, and they don't always make sense to people who are living the crisis.

Sometimes rules are there in order to protect people's rights, though they may not feel that way in your particular situation. Luckily, there are people to help you navigate the legal system and make sure you have what you need. Those people are social workers, and they're in every hospital.

Find the Helpers

Remember how Mr. Rogers always told kids to look for the helpers during a crisis, pointing out that there are always good people who dive in and do the hard work of making things right again? Your hospital (or even your aphasia clinic) has those types of helpers, and they're called social workers or patient advocates.

But how do you find them? When it comes to hospitals, you need to ask for a case manager if one isn't automatically assigned to you. Anyone on the medical team can point you to a case manager in the hospital who is specifically there to help you advocate for your loved one and navigate the system.

Your case manager can connect you with resources both inside and outside of the hospital that will help you with your caregiving responsibilities. They can connect you with the financial department in the hospital to navigate the cost of treatment. And they can tell you about any available assistance programs.

They know the system inside and out, and they can save you a lot of time when trying to get things accomplished. Beyond that, they are also there for you emotionally, as someone who has your back while you have your loved one's back.

Case managers in the hospital are included in your treatment plan, but there are also private patient advocates that can be hired and paid for by the individual. If you have the financial resources, you can hire someone to help you make sense of the paperwork and speak up on your behalf. A quick Google search for patient advocates in your area can connect you to individuals who do this work.

Find Your Voice

Listen, it's nerve-wracking to speak up for yourself when you don't like your order at a restaurant. Multiply that by 50 and it scratches the surface of how overwhelmed you may be feeling right now in being your loved one's voice when it comes to a medical situation.

You can find confidence, or at least fake-it-until-you-make-it, by practicing conversations before you need to have them. Sometimes saying the words aloud a few times can help you feel confident in what you need to say.

The reality is the squeaky wheel gets the grease, so be the squeaky wheel. You already know what needs to get done because you've been writing down action items in your caregiver journal. Be proactive. You don't need to be rude but you do need to be direct, and follow up with people to make sure things get done.

Being proactive also means finding out what the insurance company requires and keeping records. Remember your notebook and folder from the last chapter? All of the notes from phone calls to the insurance company go in your notebook, and papers go in your folder. Don't wait for your insurance company to deny a claim or let you know you're responsible for a payment you weren't counting on. From day one, you need to reach out to your insurance agent and make sure you're doing everything according to the rules. Some insurance companies have patient advocates to help you wind your way through the confusing paperwork.

It's also okay to start each conversation with a new person, or each follow-up conversation, by stating your reason for asking so many questions ahead of time. Let them know that you're trying to stave off problems by asking questions now. By putting this out there, you sometimes help the other person think through what-ifs and volunteer even more helpful information that can save you time in the future. Always work from the assumption that everyone wants to help you if they know how they can best help.

Finally, thank yous go a long way in turning those helpers you meet into partners who will guide you along the path. Everyone likes to hear that they were helpful, and often hearing those words makes people likely to help again. We have heard of many caregivers who bring cookies or treats to the people who have helped them: the therapists, nurses, and doctors. But also the receptionists and other support staff who are instrumental in supporting the care. Say thank you to the person, but also let supervisors know how someone helped you in your journey by sending a note. You never know when you'll need another favor or more information, and those small moments of kindness can bring you company as you walk the caregiving path.

Once you've found your voice it's time for the most important job you can do as a caregiver: become a question-asker-extraordinaire.

CHAPTER 6: HOW TO BE A GOOD QUESTION ASKER (AND ANSWER KEEPER)

Knowing the right questions is a skill, and it's one that all caregivers are expected to suddenly acquire the moment they enter their role. But how can you learn to be an expert question asker? This chapter will help you not only to know how to ask questions so you can gather information but also record the answers so you can find them again.

Use Your Tools

You have your caregiver journal, right? (See Chapter 4) Well, use it! Your caregiver journal is the perfect place to drop every question that pops into your brain—from the ones that come up while you're sitting by your loved one's side to the ones that slink into your head at 4 a.m. Just put a large question mark to the left of your question so you can scan down the page and find it easily.

Every time you ask a question, record the answer in your notebook. Ideally, you'll ask your question on the same day that you jot it down in your notebook so the answer will be close by. But sometimes you'll want to jog your memory by writing down a note such as "answer to the question from 9/3/19" so you can flip around in your book and mentally put the two pieces of information together.

Learn When to Ask

Your relationship with your loved one's doctors, nurses, or speech therapists is like any other relationship. It will take time to learn each other's patterns. Does the health specialist or speech therapist react well to getting all the questions at once instead of scattered throughout the appointment?

Questions at the end of the appointment? Questions at the beginning?

Once you know, tailor your question-asking to match the other person's style to best get the information you need.

Which means you'll need to play detective, and figure out what works for each individual. And when you don't know, ask. Tell them that you have a few questions and ask them when they'd like them to be asked. We know: asking a question about when you can ask questions is pretty meta, but once you get over the ridiculousness of the situation, you'll realize that asking questions in the best time period for the individual can be the difference between an appointment running smoothly and one that goes off the rails.

Give Them a Heads-Up

Of course, you can also give the person a heads-up. Telling people that you have questions and how many goes a long way. If you begin the appointment by telling the person that you're going to ask them three questions, you've set the expectation that three questions are coming their way. If they forget and start to leave the room, you can remind them that you still haven't gotten your questions asked and answered.

It can even help to hold up the correct amount of fingers as you tick off each question so they can anticipate how many more there are to go.

Of course, this means reducing your question list to the most urgent questions. A doctor, nurse, or speech therapist probably won't have time to answer a dozen questions. This is where writing them down ahead of time in your caregiver journal is a vital part of the process. Not only does writing them down ensure that you won't forget anything, but it gives you a chance to rank or combine questions so you address the most important ones first.

Getting Information from Reluctant Answer Givers

There will be times when health specialists or speech therapists will not be able to answer your question, either because they don't know the answer yet, or because it isn't information they're in a position to give. It can help you a lot if you inquire when they will be able to give you an answer or a person to contact who will be able to give you the information.

Some people are always in a hurry, and it's okay to politely point out your needs, too. Set up a question-asking appointment separate from the "care" appointment or ask if you can reserve the last five minutes of the next session/appointment for questions.

Some specialists may be willing to answer quick questions via email rather than using face-to-face time, so inquire which medium would be most helpful for the other person to get you the information you need.

Dealing with Information Overload (Trying to Answer Your Own Questions)

Asking a lot of questions means that you (hopefully!) get a lot of answers, which can lead to information overload. Simultaneously, when you're not getting answers from an individual, it can be tempting to turn to the Internet and try to answer your questions with a good, old-fashioned Google search.

After all, when you're desperate for answers, information overload sounds like a good problem to have. But it can feel like trying to drink from a firehose when information is coming fast and furious and you need to synthesize to make decisions. Where is the line where health information crosses from just enough to too much?

You can stave off information overload by asking your doctor or speech-language therapist for *one* recommended book or website and then stick to that single, best source. Hyperlinks make it tempting to jump from site to site, but use them to expand and better understand the information in your primary source rather than become more points on your information path.

If you need to make a decision and are gathering facts by doing a Google search, judge ahead of time how long you will need to find the necessary information. Add a few minutes as a buffer and set an egg timer. When the timer goes off, stop researching, even if you don't have an answer. Not having an answer in the allotted amount of time is a clue that the decision may be more complicated than you thought. In that case, you may want to return to a professional and have them help you narrow the scope of the decision.

When you tell the professional that you attempted to find answers on the internet but it wasn't satisfactory, it signals to the professional how important it is to you to have an answer. Most professionals would prefer to give you guidance rather than having you seek something on the internet so it could serve the purpose of engaging them in answering more thoroughly.

While it's fine to spread out your many, many, many questions to professionals—after all, that's what they're there for—you'll want to take the opposite approach and not overwhelm your loved one with dozens of questions. They're navigating aphasia, and there are tips in the next chapter that we can give you to help make communication easier for all.

CHAPTER 7: COMMUNICATION TIPS AND TOOLS

Aphasia-friendly communication can be summed up with this acrostic for the word *aphasia*:

A: **a**sk simple, direct questions

P: **p**rovide multiple communication options

H: **h**elp communicate if asked

A: **a**cknowledge frustration

S: **s**peak slowly and clearly

I: **i**f you don't understand, say so

A: **a**llow extra time

If you use these seven tips to guide your communication with your loved one, you'll find that a lot can be communicated, even when you're dealing with aphasia.

Keep Everyone in the Conversation

Aphasia can be isolating. Imagine not being able to easily convey your thoughts to your friends and family. Imagine not being able to understand what they're saying to you. Many people with aphasia report that everyone talks around them as if they aren't in the room. It's always important to make the individual with aphasia feel included.

Aphasia doesn't have to be isolating. In fact, it can go a long way for a person with aphasia to know that you're trying to help them to communicate and remain a part of the conversation.

Help friends and family understand that the old ways of communicating may not work, and they'll need to adjust in order to keep the person a part of the conversation.

Use More Than One Means of Communication

You already use more than one means of communication. As you speak, you also make gestures with your hands and use facial expressions in order to drive home your point. You should always use more than just your words, especially when communicating with someone who has aphasia. Additionally, be mindful of what you're using to communicate. Does the tool you're using—such as the telephone—limit the other signals you can be giving the person, such as seeing those gestures or facial expressions to aid in understanding? You may need to switch the medium, such as moving from phone call to video call, in order to enhance communication.

It's not just gestures and facial expressions. Other communication aids may be pictures, pantomime, combining writing/reading and speaking, pointing to keywords, or communication apps. Your speech pathologist will help you find the best methods and aids to communicate.

Pause and Listen

Conversations with someone with aphasia will take more time. It helps to go into the conversation knowing that you need to be patient, use pauses, and wait. The more you clearly convey that the other person should take their time, the better your loved one will be able to communicate. Stress increases communication difficulties, so make sure you are sending clear signals with your body language that you are patient. Silence is hard. We all have a tendency to fill quiet spaces in conversation, but it's necessary to allow this time when communicating with someone with aphasia.

Keep It Quiet

We all hear best when people speak to us at a normal volume rather than shouting, and when we hold conversations with minimal distractions. This fact is even more important when it comes to aphasia-friendly communication. Whenever possible, go somewhere quiet to speak, where you can see each other face-to-face. For example, turn off the television or music to minimize distractions. If there are multiple people in the conversation, make sure only one person speaks at a time. Finally, don't multitask while having a conversation; make sure both of you can focus on the words.

Keep It Simple

Keeping it simple doesn't disrespect the person. It means thinking through what you need to say, removing the unnecessary parts of the story or questions, and getting to the heart of the matter. Keeping sentences brief provides more moments to pause and ensure that both people are following the conversation.

Verify

You verify understanding in conversations without thinking, but aphasia-friendly communication asks that you do this consciously. Make sure that you understand what the other person is saying by repeating it or letting them know what you heard. Additionally, ask the person with aphasia to repeat back and verify they understood what you were saying. This "double-check" system makes for clear communication. For example, say, "I heard you say this. Am I right?"

Don't Pretend

You would never nod at your boss and pretend to understand the task she was asking you to do if your job was on the line. Approach aphasia-friendly communication in the same way. Do not pretend that you understand what the other person is saying if you really don't. Help the person by conveying that you want to understand, you have time to wait as they work on the message, and you have the flexibility to get creative with communication. It is much more rewarding for both people if everyone walks away from the conversation understanding each other.

Speak Directly to the Person

We instinctively know that we should always go to the source of the information when we have a question, but we sometimes forget that when a person has aphasia. Loop people with aphasia into the conversation by speaking to them directly instead of setting up moments where someone is speaking for the person with aphasia.

Ask If They Want Help

Adults with aphasia are adults, first and foremost. They have thoughts they want to convey and opinions they want to express. There will be times when they are having difficulty remembering or saying a word, and your first instinct may be to jump in and help. But it's more helpful to wait to see if they can do it without aid and to ask if they want help if you sense frustration.

Ask Yes/No Questions

When we're in a hurry, we instinctively start to phrase questions so people can give "yes" or "no" answers, as opposed to open-ended answers. For example, we're more likely to ask: "Can you complete this by noon?" instead of "When can you complete this?" Take this communication method and apply it when possible to make questions aphasia-friendly. While some questions require a longer response, others allow the person to give a head nod or thumbs-up motion in order to make feelings known.

Take Breaks

When you see someone yawn, or you get signals that they are checking out of the exchange, you know that it's time to wrap up the conversation. Respect these signals, and remember that people with aphasia often experience fatigue. It can be exhausting to have conversations when you have a communication disorder. Provide rest periods, and try to hold more complicated conversations while the person has energy.

Be a Good Host (So Others Can Be a Good Guest)

Whether you're still in the hospital or well into the future and out at social events, you're often serving as the "host," making sure that your loved one is part of the good times, too. Prepare visitors for your loved one's aphasia, giving them all of the tips above so they can jump straight into communication instead of fumbling in the dark. But even when people are prepared, they can subconsciously exclude a person with aphasia from the conversations. In these cases, you can't just be a host; you need to be the revealer, removing your loved one's invisibility and guiding the conversation back to the person with aphasia. Remember, speak with and not for the other person, and make sure other people do the same. When the conversation starts to swirl around the person with aphasia without including them, bring them in by asking, "Do you agree?" Or, "What do you think?"

Keeping People Informed

We'd be remiss if a chapter on communication tips didn't also cover how to communicate information to family and friends. Having a lot of loving people in your life is a good problem to have. All of those people want to be kept in the loop, especially while your loved one is still in the hospital, but also afterward when they're continuing to navigate aphasia.

Of course, you also have limited time and don't want to answer the same questions over and over again. You can set up a free Google group so you can email everyone at once and you won't need to cut-and-paste a long list of addresses. You can send out a message whenever there is news and let people know that while you're touched by all the messages of support, you won't be able to respond to individual questions. Friends and family will appreciate being in the loop, but the solution won't be taxing on the caregiver.

Talking to Kids about Aphasia

Kids are great: They are expressive communicators, their vocabulary is manageable, and they are very direct. You seldom find children pretending they understand when they don't because they feel very comfortable saying "that doesn't make any sense." And they are hungry for information, so give them the information they need.

It's understandable for kids to be confused by aphasia because aphasia is also difficult for adults to understand. How do you convey that the person is still the same on the inside though they may have trouble expressing themselves verbally on the outside?

There are so many unknowns with aphasia and no one can predict the future, so stick to the facts you know in the moment. Additionally, aphasia presents differently in each individual, so make sure you only state the problems the person is currently experiencing. Explain that aphasia affects a person's ability to speak, read, and write, and that they may or may not have difficulty understanding someone else's words.

You can open your conversation about aphasia by talking about the underlying cause, such as a stroke or head injury. Make sure children can ask questions and express their fears so you can reassure them. One important point to make is that the person with aphasia is still the same person they were before experiencing communication issues. Aphasia affects the ability to speak and write but not the person's intellect.

Kids love to know how they can help, and you can give them concrete communication tips. Explain that the person may need for the child to slow down their speech, use short sentences, or repeat their words. The child also needs to understand that they need to give the other person time to form their words. Just as kids don't like it when adults speak for them, adults with aphasia want kids to give them a chance to speak their own thoughts. Of course, kids are great at tapping into their creativity and finding new ways to communicate, such as pantomime or using pictures to express ideas.

Remind your child that people get frustrated when things are hard, and while they may witness that frustration, it isn't directed at them. People with aphasia may also get tired more easily due to underlying causes or the hard work of negotiating communication issues. Knowing these two possibilities can help the child understand a moment of frustration or having to end an activity early.

Of course, if a child is seeing a person with aphasia, they're likely at home. And speaking of home, there are things you can do to make sure that you've set up a safe and supportive environment.

CHAPTER 8: EXPLAINING APHASIA TO OTHER PEOPLE

Whether your loved one is still in the hospital or currently at home, worries about safety may be at the forefront of your mind. The world is difficult enough to navigate when all is going well, but what would your loved one do if they couldn't communicate when something was wrong? There are preventative measures you can take today to create safe spaces at home or while your loved one is out and about.

Sign up with Your Local Emergency Registry

Did you know that many areas have a special needs emergency registry? You can contact first responders *before* there is an emergency so they can know about your loved one's communication issues should an emergency ever arise.

The easiest way to get added to a registry is to call the non-emergency number for first responders in your area, such as the non-emergency number for the local police. They can tell you how to notify all emergency departments about your loved one's special needs so they'll have all of the necessary information in the event of an emergency, including your loved one's name and address.

Additionally, do an internet search for "special needs emergency registry" and your local or state government to see if your area has a broader list. For example, the Rhode Island registry covers anyone in the state of Rhode Island in case a unit from a neighboring town responds to a call.

Hopefully, your loved one will never need a first responder, but giving out this information beforehand will make things easier if an emergency ever pops up. Plus, it can bring you peace of mind.

Information Cards and Sheets

Provide your loved one with a laminated aphasia card that provides necessary information. This simple card should have a quick explanation of aphasia on one side and tips and information on the other. For example, this card can be downloaded, filled out, and laminated. (You can find it on aphasia.org under helpful resources.)

FRONT:

I HAVE APHASIA

Aphasia is a communication disorder that affects a person's ability to understand, produce, or read written or spoken words. Aphasia presents differently in each person.

In fact, the only thing everyone with aphasia has in common is that aphasia does not affect the person's intellect.

Aphasia can occur after a head injury or stroke. It can also be the result of a brain tumor. In rare cases, aphasia is the result of primary progressive aphasia (PPA), which is a neurodegenerative disorder.

FLIP CARD OVER FOR MORE INFORMATION

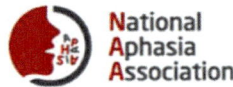
National Aphasia Association

BACK:

THE APHASIA CAREGIVER GUIDE

I HAVE APHASIA

My name is _____.

Please contact _____ in case of an emergency. You can reach them at this number: _____.

Please keep your sentences short and simple. Give me time to think and respond. I can give you a thumbs up (yes) or thumbs down (no) sign in response to yes/no questions. Verify that we both understand what the other person is saying.

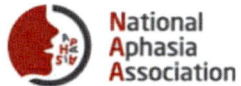
National Aphasia Association

Similarly, a one-sheet should be filled out and posted in the house with instructions for any emergency responders or even neighbors who are stopping by to be helpful. Have the page convey everything that visitors need to know about communicating with your loved one. We've provided a sample one-sheet that you can tailor to your needs in Appendix II.

Or you can make your own. Start with a quick paragraph explaining aphasia and then provide communication tips for the other person. You can give answers to common questions on the sheet so your loved one can point to the answer.

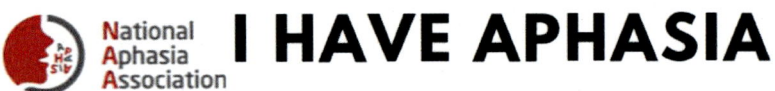

Aphasia is a communication disorder that affects a person's ability to understand, produce, or read written or spoken words. Aphasia presents differently in each person.

In fact, the only thing everyone with aphasia has in common is that aphasia does not affect the person's intellect.

Aphasia can occur after a head injury or stroke. It can also be the result of a brain tumor. In rare cases, aphasia is the result of primary progressive aphasia (PPA), which is a neurodegenerative disorder.

1 COMMUNICATION TIPS

Please keep your sentences short and simple. Give me time to think and respond. I can give you a thumbs up (yes) or thumbs down (no) sign in response to yes/no questions. Verify that we both understand what the other person is saying.

2 PLEASE CONTACT

In case of an emergency, or if I'm unable to respond, please contact _____ at this phone number: _____.

3 OTHER INFORMATION

Add additional information specific to your loved one's situation or home.

Regaining Independence

Depending on where you are in your journey, it might be hard to imagine your loved one returning to independence. Will they need you forever now that they have aphasia? The short answer is yes... and no. For most people with aphasia, what they really want is to re-establish their role in the family and community.

Even though we have many suggestions to help with support, above all else, they need you to be their friend, spouse, child, parent, sibling. Your role is not to always protect your loved one, your role is to enable them to be independent. It is impossible to predict and prevent every difficult occurrence, and sometimes you need to let go and allow them to discover their own successes and failures, sharing in the success or commiserating with the failure as a partner in this journey. Below are a few suggestions for ways to support independence.

The point of the cards and one-pagers is to help you think through which questions may come up or what information may need to be conveyed *before* a communication breakdown happens. We hope this chapter starts the wheels turning inside your brain, and you begin to see how much communication can be predicted beforehand and how support can be put in place to help your loved one regain their independence.

For example, you might consider looking at menus before you go to a restaurant so your loved one can be autonomous by choosing their meal in a low-stress environment and practicing saying what they want aloud. (Or, in some cases, writing it down so they can present their order in writing.) You may want to look ahead at outings and predict what questions may need to be asked or answers that need to be given while your loved one is out and about.

And you may want to provide your loved one with tools (such as cards or written answers) and practice so they can be independent once again. The way your loved one once communicated may have changed, but at the same time, new ways of communication have begun. You will need to shift your mindset and get creative.

We have one last chapter that deals with the financial side of aphasia. You have definitely been thrust into the role of caregiver, but you may have also been thrust into the role of breadwinner. We'll walk you through some tips to consider if you are a working-outside-the-home caregiver.

CHAPTER 9: FINANCIAL REALITIES OF APHASIA

It probably wasn't your first or second thought after you discovered your loved one was dealing with aphasia, but at some point, the financial side of life raised its hand and said, "What about me?" If you're currently working, you may be wondering how you'll make the time and space to return to your job. If you're not currently working, you may be wondering if you will need to return to the workforce and how you can make that happen, especially when your loved one clearly needs you. This chapter will give you some ideas on how to deal with these issues.

Communicate with Your Boss

When disaster strikes, such as brain trauma or stroke, or even after a less sudden diagnosis, such as primary progressive aphasia, our instinct is to notify family and friends. But add your boss or your loved one's boss to the list.

You are more likely to encounter understanding if you are proactive and communicate your needs and your loved one's situation. Start by not making assumptions. Even if this boss has not been understanding in the past, they may surprise you during your current situation. And if this boss has been supportive and nurturing, don't take their kindness for granted. Keep them in the loop. Good communication goes a long way in building understanding.

As you move through the process be sure to keep a written record. This may be as simple as writing an email after a call or meeting, thanking the person for understanding and noting everything that was agreed upon in order to verify that you're both on the same page. Aphasia is a long-term situation, and you cannot count on people remembering things they promised weeks down the line. Better to get it down so you can jog someone's memory or check your own notes in the future.

If this is your loved one's job, your primary responsibility is being reachable, answering questions when possible, and establishing ongoing communication to keep the employer in the loop.

The rest of our advice focuses on *your* work life. This is the time for you to state exactly what you need in order to do your job while also being there for your loved one. Can you get extensions on big projects, do your job remotely, or return to your job after a short leave of absence? These are all viable options to be negotiated with your employer in order to remain employed while caring for your loved one.

Where to Work

Look around the waiting room and we're sure you will see other people tending to work tasks while their loved one rests or is engaged in therapy. While hospitals generally don't have a lot of unused space, nurses may know about quiet or less-trafficked spaces on the grounds so you can take care of work-related tasks or attend meetings via a video link.

If you're having trouble concentrating, use the Pomodoro Technique developed by Francesco Cirillo to keep tabs on your loved one while still accomplishing work. Set a timer for 25 minutes and focus on work. When the timer goes off, check on your loved one for five minutes and use the break to recharge and give yourself peace of mind. Return to work for another 25 minutes, using every fourth work-break combo for one longer 15 - 20 minute break for yourself. It's easier to work in short bursts and drive all other distractions out of your mind knowing that you've built in time to check on your break, and you'll still get a little time to recharge, too. Of course, this technique only works when your loved one can entertain themselves for stretches of time or when they are engaged in an activity with another person. This presents even more reason to get help from other people when you can.

A Little Help from Your Friends

We'll talk about creating support circles in a later chapter, but this is a time to get started thinking about other people who can relieve you to do work while entertaining your loved one. While you may feel like you need to be by their side every second of the day, reality often gets in the way. Most people need to keep working, even through a loved one's health crisis. Friends and family do want to help and will tell you to "call them if you need them." Well, you need them, so call them, and ask them to help with this specific area of need.

Ask friends and family to set up a schedule that gives you specific work time frames so you can let your employer know when you'll be able to complete work-related tasks. So many jobs require us to be always available; that can be tricky when you add a complex caregiving layer to your schedule. Some people are able to set up "office hours" or set times when certain colleagues know they can reach you. Knowing you have a set work time in your schedule can help you look ahead and focus in order to use the time effectively.

Moreover, you will need to set up a care situation when you're out of the hospital. (Or, if you're already out of the hospital, you can set it up now.) Making sure you have the time and space to work while your loved one is spending time with other family members or friends is an important part of tackling money matters when it comes to living with aphasia.

Getting a Job

It can be overwhelming to think about returning to (or starting in) the workforce if you've been out for a while, but don't let fears derail your life. If you need to get a job, take the first step by creating or updating your resume. If you've been out of the workforce for a while, you may want to create a skills-based resume. A quick Google search for "skills-based resume" will show you plenty of examples. Consider the skills necessary for the type of job you want to get, and then detail the work you have done to develop those skills. Think back through your day-to-day life and recent volunteer work, and sell yourself.

While most jobs still require a person to show up in a brick-and-mortar office or workplace, there are also plenty of remote-only positions. Flexjobs (https://www.flexjobs.com) is a paid site that allows you to search for remote-only or part-time work in your area. Other free job boards, including Indeed, Monster, or Glassdoor all provide ways to use telecommute-only as a search term.

Working Guilt

You may feel guilty wanting to take care of work tasks rather than spend time with your loved one. That's understandable and will need to be overcome. Your loved one needs to work at improving communication skills, but you need to work to earn money so you can afford basic needs as well as medical care. You both have work roles to play.

Working can give you a much-needed break from constant caregiving, which is exhausting. Having a daily reminder of normal life coupled with feeling effective at work can help to combat the emotional drain that comes from living with aphasia. Never feel guilty for wanting to spend time in a situation that is under your control. It can help you gather energy so you can get through the times that are outside your control.

Payment for Therapy

Healthcare in America is in constant flux, so we cannot go into the specifics of insurance plans or Medicare/Medicaid. Instead, we're going to direct you to resources on the web, such as ASHA's frequently asked questions about using Medicaid to pay for speech therapy. The Affordable Care Act created ten essential health benefits (EHB) that all insurance plans need to cover. One of the ten EHB points is coverage of "rehabilitative and habilitative services and devices," which includes speech therapy.

But not all therapists are covered by insurance or Medicare/Medicaid. *Before* you get speech therapy, you need to ensure your provider can bill Medicare/Medicaid for speech services or your insurance plan accepts the provider. The case manager at the hospital can help you connect with providers who accept Medicare/Medicaid or your insurance plan.

For reimbursed coverage through private insurance or Medicare/Medicaid situations, you will need a script from the doctor for speech pathology services. Make sure you get this referral *before* you set up any appointments.

The Centers for Medicare and Medicaid Services site also has individual state plans. Make sure you look at your specific state to learn which services are offered in your area.

Also ask to have meetings with a case manager at the hospital, a member of the billing department, or the financial department of your speech therapy center. In all cases, the people working in these jobs will be able to tell you about resources in your area or set up payment plans so you can afford services.

The financial realities of aphasia can sting, but they're just one source of stress you're feeling at the moment. The next section of this booklet contains helpful advice on navigating other feelings that accompany aphasia: from finding calm in the stormy sea of emotion to finding joy again in your new normal. The rest of this booklet focuses on *you*, the caregiver. In other words, while you're looking out for your loved one, we're looking out for you.

CHAPTER 10: FINDING CALM ON THE STORMY SEAS

We're not starting with "finding calm" because aphasia is all doom and gloom, but because aphasia is stressful, both for the people with aphasia and the people who love them. This chapter is really the equivalent of securing your own oxygen mask before helping others. You can't be the best caregiver you can be if you're struggling with your own unmet emotional needs. So we'll start with two facts: (1) there is an emotional side of aphasia and (2) there are things you can do to address that emotional side that are worth doing because it will make you a better caregiver.

Finding Empathy

It can be difficult to be empathetic when you're in a stressful situation. It can be difficult to remain patient with your loved one when the progress is slow or not at all. It can be difficult to remain patient with doctors, nurses, and therapists when you feel like they're not hearing you or meeting your needs.

The first step is acknowledging this. There is nothing wrong with you if you're finding aphasia difficult to navigate emotionally. Wait, let's say it again, a little louder.

There is nothing wrong with you.

Hopefully, you feel a little bit better knowing that everyone struggles with caregiving, and there is nothing wrong with that. The rest of this chapter will walk through ways you can make things emotionally easier on yourself so you can focus on moving forward.

Switch Your Perspective

The first thing you might try is a little mind shift. When you feel yourself getting frustrated, excuse yourself from the situation for a moment, and consider everything from the other person's point of view. Shifting your perspective can help you realize that the person isn't intentionally trying to frustrate you or ruin your day. They might just be just distracted, not understanding, or being pulled in too many directions, just like you are.

Sometimes this moment is all you need to get a hold of your emotions and return to the conversation, acknowledging the other person's perspective while also conveying your own. We cannot always get inside the mind of another person and understand why they're doing what they're doing; it might help to remember writer Ian MacLaren's wise words: "Be kind, for everyone you meet is fighting a hard battle." By imagining someone else's backstory, you stop seeing them as an obstacle and instead as a fellow traveler who will respond better when offered kindness.

Switch Your Timeline

Aphasia takes the Gregorian calendar and twists it around. November becomes March and "soon" becomes "two weeks from now." If you are someone accustomed to seeing progress proportionate to effort expended, you need to shift your thinking and slow down. You're now on aphasia time.

Everything will take longer than you think. It will take longer than you want to get a referral, make an appointment, and have those big wins as your loved one finds new ways to communicate. Knowing this can help you adjust your expectations. Slow down and embrace aphasia time. Truly, when it comes to aphasia, things can potentially take a long time. It will help you focus on what is important and tune everything else out.

Do Breathing Exercises

The military teaches its members how to do combat tactical breathing or CTB. While you're clearly not on an actual battlefield, you are on a figurative one. This breathing technique can be done anywhere, at any time, and it can help you slow down your body and mind.

Become friends with the number four: breathe in to the count of four, hold your breath to the count of four, exhale to the count of four, and again hold your breath to the count of four. Then start all over. In fact, it can help to think about traveling the perimeter of a square while you move through each section of this breathing technique. Every five "breathing squares" equal one minute. Aim to complete ten breathing squares when you're trying to calm yourself down and unwind from a stressful moment.

Take a Five-Minute Vacation

The irony is that you can't leave to take a vacation right at the moment of life when you most need a vacation! After all, your loved one needs you here. But we suggest you start building five-minute vacations into your day and going on them regularly.

Just like a real vacation, you need to schedule and plan for a five-minute vacation or you won't make the time in your busy day. Start by making a list of ten simple things you enjoy. It can be anything from a cup of tea or a square of chocolate to reading a chapter in a book.

Now break down these favorite things into five-minute moments and literally schedule them into your day by making an appointment on your calendar. You may want to schedule your first thing in the morning to ensure that you take five minutes for yourself before you dive into helping other people, another at a midway point in the day to serve as a break, and another before bed so you have something to look forward to during hard moments in the day.

When you are on one of your vacations, set aside all other thoughts and worries. We promise, they will be waiting for you when you return from your mini-vacation. But while you're on vacation, don't look at your phone, don't multitask and try to do something more productive, and certainly don't think about your to-do list or the needs of your loved one. This is YOU time, and you need it in order to recharge and be your best self.

We will get into other ways you can take care of yourself in Chapter 13, including eating nutritious meals and working in a little exercise, but we wanted to kick off this section by providing you with a few quick coping mechanisms when the emotions of living with aphasia threaten to pull you under. This is a long journey, and leaning on other people will make it easier. We'll help you set up some support systems and set them in motion before we return to taking care of *you* on a deeper level.

CHAPTER 11: FINDING YOUR CIRCLES OF SUPPORT

The Beatles touched on something important when they sang about getting a little help from their friends. Everyone needs a support system, but it's even more important when your emotional resources are being quickly drained as a caregiver. This chapter will help you find your circle of support and learn how to delegate like a pro, even if your friends and family live far away.

Creative Problem Solving

Open your notebook and write down a time when you had a problem and came up with a brilliant solution. It can be as small as that time you skillfully covered up a stain to as large as a plan you executed at work that became a major success.

We want you to write this down because you now have written proof that you can tackle problems, big and small. You're a creative problem solver, and caregiving is the Olympics of creative problem solving. Problems will pop up every day, and you will need to be the person with the plan. Anytime you feel overwhelmed, turn to this page in your journal and remember: you can do it.

But it's also a place where you can begin to think about the importance of circles of support. Look back at your creative problem solving win. Who else was there? Who helped you along the way? Be as specific as possible. We're not going to ask you to return to these people now, but noticing them is an important step.

The first rule of creative problem solving is never going it alone. You need a team––the bigger the better. Some people on your team you already know. They are the doctors, nurses, speech therapists, and social workers. They are your friends, family, neighbors, and community members. Others you'll meet along the way, especially when you set up your circles of support. You'll quickly learn that there are a lot of people out there you can count on, even if you can't imagine your circles of support yet.

Draw a Circle

Return to your journal and write your loved one's name in the center of the circle. Put your name—or if you're not the primary caregiver, write the name of the primary caregiver—on ring one, surrounding the person with aphasia. The primary caregiver is the person with aphasia's first circle of support.

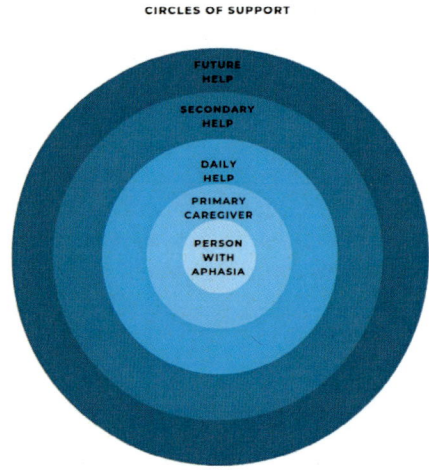

CIRCLES OF SUPPORT

Now it's time to support the caregiver. These are the people closest to the caregiver, who can provide daily help, sometimes before being asked. These are the people you can count on to be there on a day-to-day basis. They may be close friends and family, professionals, or hired help. They are the people who can run errands for the caregiver or provide a valuable break. They also provide integral services such as therapy.

The next circle of support are the people who will step up when asked. They are more distant friends and family, but also include community members and peripheral friends. These are the people who are concerned when they hear about your loved one and ask how they can help. Don't dismiss their offers; we'll talk about how to loop these people in to make your life easier in a moment. In the meantime, put them in the next ring.

You may want to add another ring after that of future support people: people that you could turn to in the future. They are resources in your community that provide support, people you can go to for answers, or people who may be able to provide a favor down the road. You may never need to use this circle of support, but it can be empowering to think about all of the people out there who possibly want to help you with your caregiving.

Ring Theory

Your circle of support should feel like a hug. The primary caregiver's circle goes around the person with aphasia, the next circle supports the primary caregiver, and the circle after that provides support for the people closest to the caregiver. In each case, the surrounding circle prevents burnout when used correctly.

But those circles of support are also valuable in knowing how to *be* emotionally supportive. Susan Silk came up with her "Ring Theory" back in 2013. This theory states how support should flow during a crisis or chronic situation.

The person experiencing aphasia is the center of the ring. Their closest loved ones—the ones doing the caregiving—are the next ring. The caregiver's support system—friends, specialists, etc.—are the larger ring after that.

Knowing your ring is important because your placement in the situation dictates where you should look for empathy. As Silk explains in a *Los Angeles Times* article,

> Here are the rules. The person in the center ring can say anything she wants to anyone, anywhere. She can kvetch and complain and whine and moan and curse the heavens and say, "Life is unfair" and "Why me?" That's the one payoff for being in the center ring. Everyone else can say those things too, but only to people in larger rings.

Meaning, the caregiver shouldn't complain to the person with aphasia, though they should definitely seek empathy from people on outside rings, such as specialists and friends. And friends should be giving, not seeking, empathy from the person with aphasia or the caregiver.

Silk says the point is "comfort IN, dump OUT." This means the comfort flows toward the person with aphasia, and the complaining about the situation flows towards people on the outside of the crisis. Everyone has someone to talk to; the person with aphasia isn't asked to bear a large emotional burden, and the feelings of the people on the outer rings aren't given more weight than the people closest to the crisis.

Help or compassion also flows toward the center of the circle, to that person with aphasia in the center of the rings. This is the direction you want that compassion to flow, towards the person who needs it most. This isn't to say that your favorite nurse or speech therapist doesn't deserve a treat and thank you for their hard work, but that good energy and help needs to be directed at the person in most need.

Moreover, support networks of friends and specialists should be holding up close caregivers too. When comfort flows in, it washes over all the people as it makes its way toward the center of the circle.

Delegating like a Champ

It's now time to put your circles of support into action. There will be times that people offer to help but you don't know how to direct them, times that people don't step up to the plate at all, and times when the heavens align and the right help is delivered at the right time. Welcome to the world of delegating, an important task necessary for the survival of every caregiver. You can't do it all, and luckily, you usually don't have to.

People want to help when they know there's a problem, and it's mutually beneficial to allow them to help. They feel useful, and you get to focus your attention on your loved one with aphasia or get a much-needed break.

Notifying people that you need support is actually the second step. The first step is defining who is in that possible pool of helpers. Look at your circles of support and start organizing them into an email list. Begin with family members who will want to help, even if they live far away. (After all, even people living far away can order a meal for delivery to save you from cooking one night.)

Add your friends and your loved one's friends. You may be surprised by who steps out of the woodwork to help, so include everyone who makes sense. If you belong to any communities such as a religious organization or a social group, add those people, too. People from your circles of support are your dream team — the people who will step up and help. The magic is that you have people you know will step up and help, but there are people you're not expecting to jump to attention, and they're on that list, too. Sometimes helping brings out the best in people.

Making a List of Needs

Before you reach out to your dream team, come up with a list of tasks that would help you. There are plenty of things people will offer to do, but not all of these tasks will help. Some will require you to be home at a certain time or require you to create a long list of instructions that takes longer to assemble than doing the task itself.

This is the time to be transparent and think of tasks that others can do. Especially focus on the ones that take you away from your loved one with aphasia, but also consider tasks people can do to give you a break. If you make them a shopping list, can they go to the grocery store for you? Do a load of laundry? Walk your dog? Pick up another helper at the airport? This is a time where "good" needs to be good enough. People may not do it exactly as you would do it, but if the task gets done, consider it a win.

There are no awards for being a caregiver who does it all, so don't be embarrassed about asking for help. We all need it from time to time. Think about how good you feel when someone entrusts you with a task. Know that you're doing the same for someone else who wants to make your aphasia journey a little easier.

Using Technology

Now that you have a list and know your dream team, it's time to set up a way to communicate. This is a place where technology comes in handy.

Sites such as CaringBridge can help disseminate information and keep people informed. Lotsa Helping Hands or SignUpGenius can ensure that you have coverage and other people get reminders to do their tasks. You may want to create a Google Group so you can send out one email and have it reach many people. Or you may want to set up an email account specifically for your caregiving needs so these emails don't flood your regular inbox.

Make sure you end each email or CaringBridge post with a call-to-action. For instance, tell them exactly what you need and how you would like support. "I have an appointment for myself this week, so I would love for someone to come Thursday from 3 p.m. to 5 p.m. to be with Jim. Please email me by Tuesday evening if you're able to help with this." Being specific means that you'll get fewer questions in the long-run, and people have a sense of when you need the information and what they're committing to do.

Making a Counter Offer

Sometimes people will offer to help, but what they're offering to do won't actually be helpful. Don't turn them down entirely; make a counteroffer.

It's fine to tell someone, "Thank you so much! I don't need a meal right now, but I do need someone to go grocery shopping for me on Wednesday. If I make you a list and give you some cash, could you do that for me?" They may say no, but more likely, their first offer was made because they thought it was something you'd want. Once they hear what you actually need, they're likely to change course and do your idea instead.

Remember, you don't need to take all the help that is offered, but it is in your best interest to give tasks to all interested parties.

When No One Steps Up

Sometimes no one will step up. Sometimes you'll need to let go of expectations and be okay with the fact that dinner is cereal again and the laundry didn't get done. Life will go on, and taking care of yourself and your loved one is more important than a clean house.

You may also have people flake on tasks because they volunteer to help without knowing what they're getting themselves into, or they may have good intentions and then forget. Be forgiving; everyone makes mistakes and you don't know what is happening in someone else's life. If your circle of support is tight, you may be able to quickly get another volunteer if your first one drops out. If you notice someone is a super-helper, you may even ask them if you can use them as a safety net if other people fall through.

If it's financially feasible, consider hiring support; either to supplement or in place of friends. There are grocery delivery services, cleaning services, and restaurants that drop off meals. You can schedule these time-savers around your schedule.

Getting by with a Little Help from Your Friends

Look back at that first major win that you wrote in your journal, and then look at the circles of support that you've amassed. Being able to put together support is one of the key tasks of a caregiver, and you just knocked it out of the park. If the Beatles were here, they'd join you in a rousing chorus from their song.

Whenever you get overwhelmed, turn back to these lists and remember that you have exceptional leadership skills. You're leading the way forward, helping your loved one by helping yourself. A medical crisis that leads to aphasia can bring people together just as much as it can sever loose friendship ties. In the next chapter, we'll take a look at the wins and losses that can occur in friendships when you start utilizing those circles of support.

CHAPTER 12: YOU'VE DELEGATED... NOW WHAT?

You've created your circles of support and sent out an email asking for help. Now what? The answers that are pouring in (or not pouring in) may be filling you with feelings. More is not always merrier, even when you're grateful to have people helping you with your new normal. And the other reality is that it can sting to not hear from close friends and family when you're in a crisis. This chapter will help you learn how to lean on friends and family, understand the people who don't step forward, and navigate having people in your space.

Get a Super-Helper

Have you ever seen a Hanukkah menorah? Hanukkah is a Jewish holiday that lasts for eight nights, and a single candle is lit for each of those eight nights. But the menorah has nine spots. What's up with that?

The answer is that the ninth spot, usually placed slightly higher than the other eight spots, is held for the shammash candle. This candle isn't a Hanukkah candle; It's a helper candle whose sole job is to light the other candles and help them perform their nightly task. It's there in case one of the main candles burns out and needs to be relit. Think of it as the overseer candle that makes sure all the other candles can perform their job well.

Every caregiver needs their own human shammash.

You have a list of caring people, eager to help. Look down that list and see if there is someone more eager, more organized, more emotionally supportive than the others. Designate this person to be your human shammash. Their key job is to light the action by coordinating the help, making sure people have the information or support they need to do their task, and stepping in whenever a helper gets burned out or doesn't show up.

The super-helper may not be the obvious choice. Someone close to you may not be the right person for the task, while a peripheral friend may feel overjoyed to be given such an important job.

Contact your super-helper *first*; lining up this position is critical. Once you have this person in place, you should be able to hand them your tasks and calendar (what things you need done and when) and they will do the rest. Make sure you ask them how they want people to contact them as they coordinate errands, meals, and breaks, and then let the rest of the list know about this point of contact. Once this person is in place, you should only need to deal with a single person to ensure that everything gets done.

Make sure you check in often with your coordinator and let them know how much you appreciate their help. They may not feel like they're doing a lot by responding to emails and sending out shopping lists, just as the shammash candle may not feel like it's as important as the candles that mark the nights of the holiday. But the reality is that caregiving delegation cannot run smoothly without this person, making them the most important helper on your team and the true heavy-lifter taking the weight off your shoulders.

List of Needs and Non-Delegation

Remember that list of needs from Chapter 11? It's time to make a corresponding list of non-delegated tasks. These are the things that you never want to have anyone else do. This list will be different for each person.

Once you've completed your list of tasks you—and only you—can do, take one more look and be realistic. Are these all things that really and truly need your presence to go smoothly or make you comfortable? If you can remove anything from your list, take it off your list. Once you have your list set, understand that these tasks are the only things *you* must get done. Feel okay about delegating all other tasks or letting things go for a bit.

Remember, there are no awards for being the caregiver who does it all, and there is no shame if your list of non-delegated tasks only contains two or three "no go" items that you keep for yourself. It doesn't mean that you won't do anything else; it just means that you've ranked what is most important for you to do first and foremost, an important boundary for every caregiver.

Turn over the rest of the list of delegatable tasks to your super-helper and let them get the schedule in place.

What to Do about Not-So-Friendly Friends

You have a super-helper, you have support systems, and you have your own boundaries. In all three cases, you have people taking action, making sure the world keeps spinning. But what do you do with the people you expected to come to your aid who are nowhere to be seen, or, even worse, tell you that they'll be there to help out and then don't follow through on their promises?

We touched on this in Chapter 11 just to introduce the idea, but it's worth exploring because everyone experiences a letdown or two while caregiving. It may seem like someone else has everyone jumping to their aid while you flounder in rough times, but truly, *everyone* has a story of the person who didn't show up or didn't reach out.

Health crises open up a lot of feelings in other people. It is *not* your job to manage their feelings or assuage their fears. (Remember Chapter 11? Comfort IN and dump OUT.) But we offer this as an explanation for why people sometimes disappear right when you need them most. Aphasia makes some people uncomfortable. The underlying causes for the aphasia make people worried. And some people buckle under tremendous internal pressure to say or do the right thing. Doing nothing is sometimes a sign that the person is behaving like a deer in headlights more than a terrible person ignoring your needs. Remember, this is usually more about *them* than it is about you or your loved one.

Before you feel hurt, look back at how much information you've conveyed. Some people aren't aware that there is a problem (no matter how clear it is for those living it) without spelling it out for them. They may not understand aphasia and how it affects your loved one's life. Send them to the NAA website and help them understand what is going on so they know your dire need for help to go from moment to moment. Remember, if it's months after the initial crisis and you're living your day-to-day life, family and friends may not have a strong understanding of how aphasia affects your world without spelling it out for them.

In the end, if they *do* understand what is going on and are still frozen and not giving help, you can bring them out of the figurative headlights by letting them know that even small tasks help. Release them from needing to say or do the "right" thing by telling them how they can support you in no uncertain terms. Let them know how much you've appreciated their help in the past.

Again, remember that this is about *them*. And you do not have the time or energy to waste on holding grudges or tallying up help. Focus on the people who are there for you and know that the people who aren't there for you may have reasons that you would find understandable if you were hearing about them in a story rather than living the effects in the moment. Consider that, and let those people go, knowing that they may step up in the future or have shown their true colors as individuals in your life. It can be good for your soul to forgive and forget, releasing yourself from feeling frustrated and hurt.

If you don't have people stepping up or, even worse, flaking out and not keeping their promise, it's time to hire support. Yes, it's out there, and some of it is even funded.

Hiring Help

Even if you have friends and family stepping up, you may want to hire people to do some of the day-to-day tasks. You don't need to reinvent the wheel, these services already exist and are there to fulfill your needs.

Consider starting with something basic and concrete: a grocery delivery service. Most grocery stores have their own proprietary service that either bags your ordered groceries for curbside pickup or delivers groceries straight to your home. Do an internet search for your local grocery store or the largest chain store in your area and see if they have a service already in place.

Beyond the service connected with your local establishment, there are national services—such as Target or Amazon—that can mail non-perishables to your home. Consider getting basics delivered so you don't have to worry about hitting the grocery store on your way home from a speech therapy appointment.

Next, Googling "errand services" + "your area" will bring you to a world of localized help that you can hire to do everything from drive to appointments to pick up dry cleaning. For instance, A Second Me, a service out of Virginia, can help with day-to-day tasks such as making appointments or organizing claims. They can also help with returning library books or ordering prescriptions.

If you don't find an errand service in your area, turn to your town listserv and post a call-for-help, asking if you can hire someone for a few hours a week to help with tasks. There are usually stay-at-home parents or students who are happy to take the job. You can find your town listserv on sites such as Nextdoor (https://nextdoor.com) or by searching for your area in Google groups (https://groups.google.com/). You can also turn to sites such as TaskRabbit (https://www.taskrabbit.com) to find people looking for quick, simple jobs.

Caregiver Relief Funds

Not all help is paid help. According to the website for The National Family Caregiver Support Program (NFCSP), their role is to provide "grants to states and territories to fund various supports that help family and informal caregivers care for older adults in their homes for as long as possible." Their website (https://acl.gov/programs/support-caregivers/national-family-caregiver-support-program) contains resources for caregivers to tap into this support.

Moreover, there are local and national Caregiver Relief Funds. Make sure that you are using a legitimate service—you should not be asked to pay a fee or give a lot of personal information in order to qualify for help—and check the Family Caregiver Alliance (https://www.caregiver.org/) for vetted resources. You can also do a search for "caregiver relief fund" + "your state" to find localized versions of national resources.

These relief funds aren't here to fund or cover the medical part of caregiving; they don't, for instance, cover speech therapy. But they *do* provide valuable help for a short period of time that can make your life easier. These services may send someone to run errands or provide you with a break.

And speaking of breaks, there are also adult daycare centers that can provide relief for caregivers, and many are well-versed in aphasia. A Google search for "adult daycare center" + "your area" will bring you listings to these programs that provide a safe space providing care while giving you a few hours to take care of errands, work, or have a break.

If you call the center, they'll be able to tell you what services they provide for people with aphasia. ARCH, the National Respite Network and Resource Center, has an excellent overview of adult daycare and how to find a center (https://archrespite.org/images/docs/Factsheets/fs_54-adult_day_care.pdf).

Navigating Help

As much as it's wonderful to have help at your fingertips, we'd be remiss if we didn't also admit that having help is hard. No matter how helpful the help is, having a stranger in your home or feeling the need to entertain or make small talk with your volunteering family and friends can feel like a burden. It can often add stress just as much as it relieves it.

After all, people want their home to be a harbor, and it's hard to feel like a rest space if you have people milling about or if you're on-guard, waiting for a grocery delivery.

It can help to focus on the positives over the negatives. Yes, you need to give up five minutes of your day making small talk, but you gained a half-hour of cooking time because your nephew dropped off a meal. Or you have people moving your magazines to the wrong table, but those very same people are giving you a two-hour window to go to your own appointments.

Those connections can also be a time when you remind yourself that every person walking over your threshold, making a phone call, or sending an email are all cheering you on. They are there not to irritate you but because they love you and want to be helpful.

Be Your Own Helper

Remember how we kicked off this chapter talking about designating a super-helper who will guide the help coordination? There's a larger point to this person. Caregiving is about delegating because the caregiver has needs, too. Your needs don't disappear just because your loved one has greater, immediate needs. If you don't tend to your needs, what you end up with is a caregiver down for the count.

The next chapter will address your daily needs—from getting enough sleep to putting the best foods in your body. Caregivers need to make self-care a priority if they want to be the best caregiver they can be. And we know that describes you.

CHAPTER 13: CARE FOR THE CAREGIVER

You are important, too. That fact may get lost in the day-to-day stress of helping your loved one navigate aphasia, but we want you to know that we hear you and see you and applaud you. We hope that *you* take five minutes out of every day to do the same thing, recognizing the important job you're doing as a caregiver.

One way you can show that gratitude towards yourself is to practice self-care. Like delegation, this is one of the most important tasks of a caregiver. This chapter will walk you through the places where you may not be focusing enough on your own needs to provide tips for getting yourself back on track.

What Is Self-Care?

Self-care is pretty simple—it's everything you do to put yourself first and ensure that your basic needs are met. Those needs include eating, sleeping, exercise, and general stress relief. While the word may conjure up a vision of bubble baths and scented candles (and there is nothing wrong with bubble baths and scented candles if they help you relax), it is an essential part of caregiving. You cannot take care of someone else if you're not taking care of yourself.

Your loved one is the center of your world right now because they have enormous needs. But think about it—humans are accustomed to being the center of their own world for good reason. It takes a lot of work to keep a human being going. So the point of self-care is to create a reminder that you matter, too. You cannot allow core elements of your life to fall to the wayside if you want to be an effective caregiver.

Which means you need to create a no-guilt-zone. No, we're not talking about literally setting up fences and hanging a sign that reads "No Guilt," but we are talking about making a list of things you need to do every day to keep yourself healthy and checking off those things when you do them.

So without further ado, open your caregiver notebook and write Self-Care at the top of the page. Now write down "Eating" and underneath that, "three meals plus snacks."

Eating

Three meals + snacks

Underneath that, write "sleeping" and the number of hours you need to sleep to feel your best. Think about the time you need to wake up (or the time you naturally wake up) and work backward eight or so hours from your daily start time. That is your bedtime.

Sleeping
8 hours—from 10 p.m. to 6 a.m.

Write down a form of exercise you enjoy or can work into your day. If you can't do it daily, try for three times per week. No excuses: you don't need to hit the gym. You can take a walk around the speech therapy clinic, practice chair yoga, or do a seven-minute workout via an app. We'll talk more about that below.

Exercise
Walk around the speech therapy clinic three times per week

Finally, create a list of at least five things that make you happy that you can do on a daily basis. Playing with grandchildren, traveling to favorite places, and getting a massage may all be favorite things, but they're not small things you can do to relax on a daily basis. The point is to focus on yourself. So think about things you like to do that take ten minutes or so. Start listing as many as possible. You're going to choose one thing from this list to do every day.

Me Time
Play solitaire
Read a chapter in my book
Watch videos on YouTube
Video chat with my friend
Read a magazine
Eat a few squares of dark chocolate

You now have the start of your self-care list. Check this page daily to get in the habit of continuously addressing these four areas of self-care. Let's dive deeper into each category to make sure you're taking care of yourself.

Eating

Not all food is created equally. It's not just *if* you're putting food in your mouth. It's *what* you're putting in your mouth. Food doesn't just taste good; it's fuel. So while you need calories to "go," you need vitamins, minerals, protein, and carbohydrates to stay healthy.

When you're stressed out, it's difficult to eat well. You may be eating meals in waiting rooms or spending long hours out of the house. Moreover, comfort food is…….. comforting, even if that comfort food often isn't very healthy. There will be times when you won't be able to avoid the vending machine lunch or the fast food dinner, but those should be rare days. Let people in your circle of support know that it would be helpful to receive prepared meals—preferably individual portions that you can freeze and heat up during the week rather than a single, large meal.

Planning ahead ensures that you have proper nutrition. Make sure you have basic staples stocked in your house that can be turned into a healthy meal in little or no time. Place frozen vegetables in your freezer so you can heat up a single serving with each meal or a bag of baby carrots you can snack on while you cook. Yogurt smoothies that come prepared in the dairy section are a great grab-and-go option for a quick protein fix. Even milk and a healthy cereal are better than junk food grabbed out of a hospital vending machine.

Create a food bag that you take with you as a walking, portable pantry. Lärabars and other protein bars may not be the pinnacle of nutrition, but they'll fill your belly and keep you from grabbing a candy bar. Nuts, dried fruit, granola, and pretzels can all be kept in a bag that you bring with you or leave in the car, depending on the weather. Throw an extra water bottle in the bag so you always have a drink on the go, too.

Focus on making a meal plan every Sunday for the following week with healthy, simple-to-make meals for each day. It doesn't help if you plot out ambitious, three-course dinners if you're too tired to make them at the end of the day. Aim for simple foods that are quick to fix (Google "30-minute meals" to find thousands of recipes) and save the gourmet meals for the future when you've found your footing.

Moreover, track what you eat every so often in your caregiver notebook. It will help you see patterns. For instance, are you always grabbing something unhealthy or skipping a meal on a certain day of the week due to an appointment? You can take that knowledge and plan ahead so you have something nutritious to eat on the road. Looking back at meals can also jog your memory when you can't think of what you're in the mood to eat at the moment.

We're starting with food because you need good fuel to avoid the peaks and valleys that come with poor nutrition. Plus, once you're properly fueled, you can get better sleep.

Sleeping

How many hours of sleep per day are you getting? We can guarantee you that if you're not paying attention to your sleep, the answer is usually "not enough." But sleep affects the strength of your immune system. It's a vital part of staying healthy so you can continue caregiving.

More serious though is the fact that sleep deprivation can lead to car accidents. According to the AAA Foundation for Traffic Safety, you are twice as likely to get into an accident if you get under seven hours per sleep each 24-hour period. Drowsy driving is responsible for 20% of fatal car accidents. Not sleeping is not an option. Your life––and the lives of other people on the road––are at stake.

Sleep experts recommend setting up a wind-down routine before bed. Ban screens from the bedroom as you're getting ready for bed because they can interrupt sleep. Do something relaxing for the last few minutes before you turn off the lights. Try reading, taking a bath, or listening to music to cue your body that it's time to sleep. Of course, you may be beyond exhausted and won't need a routine; it would be time better spent to just jump to the sleep. At the very least, try to keep a consistent bedtime and wake-up time so your body can find its rhythm.

It can be difficult to clear your mind of worries when you're actively caregiving, but it's vital that you mark these moments before bed as a worry-free time. All your worries will still be there in the morning. Revisit them *after* you're properly rested. In fact, once you're properly rested, you can layer in exercise, which can help clear nervous thoughts from your mind.

Exercise

Maybe they should call it care*sitting* instead of caregiving. Caregivers spend a lot of time sitting in places, waiting for their loved ones. Even once you get home and appointments fall into a manageable routine, exercise can fall by the wayside. This is a shame, because caregiving is stressful, and the adrenaline and cortisol your body produces when it's under stress can be addressed just by getting up and moving.

Exercise doesn't have to be a trip to the gym. Think of exercise as anything that gets you out of a chair and moving (or in a chair and moving). Walk around the room or building for twenty minutes, and if that's impossible, walk in place. Walk the stairs while you're waiting for a speech therapy appointment to be over. Jog the perimeter of the clinic building. Stretch while you wait in line.

Apps are your friend. Your smartphone has made it possible to take exercise classes from the comfort of your own home. There are apps for yoga, apps for a seven-minute workout, and apps that play music so you can throw an impromptu dance party for one. The point is to take a few minutes each day to move your body. Those endorphins will help decrease the negative thoughts that keep you awake at night or worry you during the day. And once you've exercised your body, you can turn towards nourishing your soul. Taking time for yourself every day is vital.

Me Time

Or really, that should be YOU time because this section is all about you. We can't give you suggestions for how you should spend your Me Time because what makes you happy is unique to each person. But creating a go-to list of simple things you can do daily that make you happy and then doing at least one of the things on the list for ten minutes ensures that even if the rest of your day is spent arguing with the insurance company, driving your loved one to speech therapy, and writing emails to update friends and family, you will have spent at least a small amount of time on yourself.

Ideally, you'd set up your day to ensure that you have at least three sessions of Me Time. Start your day with a ten-minute session so you feel energized having done something for yourself. Take a break in the middle of the day for another quick session. And end the day by using the last ten minutes before bed to do something relaxing that makes you happy.

If you're struggling to figure out things to do, you can start with meditation. Apps such as Headspace (https://www.headspace.com), Insight Timer (https://insighttimer.com), or Smiling Mind (https://www.smilingmind.com.au) can all teach you how to meditate from the comfort of your home. Adding in gentle breathing exercises––literally just breathing in for the count of four, holding it for the count of four, releasing it for the count of four, then holding it again for the count of four––can increase relaxation.

If you can activate a relaxation response, you can better deal with the stress that accompanies aphasia. By releasing that stress, you're accessing a deeper well of compassion and patience, two integral parts of caregiving. So don't look at Me Time as selfish; look at it as one more element of good caregiving.

Other Forms of Self-Care

Of course, there are other forms of self-care that you'll need to engage in when you're a caregiver. Your own medical needs can't fall by the wayside. Get your flu shot, attend doctor appointments, and take time to floss your teeth. These things matter because your loved one can't afford to have you fall apart because you're not taking care of yourself.

Know Your Boundaries

Every person has a limit to how much they can endure, emotionally and physically. Even if you are practicing self-care, you may reach a time when you hit your limit and experience burnout. Burning out means feeling overtired or over-stressed. If you wake up in the morning wondering how you're going to get through the day, you're experiencing burnout.

In those cases, you need to take a step back and get a break. We cannot say strongly enough how important it is to put yourself first for a moment when you hit a limit. If you're saying, "It's not possible!" ask yourself what would you do if you had the flu and couldn't come near your loved one. The person who you would call to take your place? Call that person now. Truly. Your health is too important.

It helps to plan your Plan B ahead of time so you know what would you do and who you would call during an emergency. Use that Plan B if you feel stressed beyond your breaking point. Remember, you are not doing your loved one any favors if you're not taking care of yourself.

Taking care of yourself also means addressing your feelings. Next time you're sitting in a waiting room, look at the people around you. All those things you're thinking and feeling are completely normal, and the people around you are thinking and feeling them too. It is a part of the highs and lows of caregiving. In the next chapter, we'll talk about that range, from the deep love to the deep frustration. So take a deep breath before diving in.

CHAPTER 14: DEALING WITH YOUR FEELINGS

According to Dacher Keltner of Berkeley's Greater Good Science Center, people experience 27 different emotions, and each of those emotions come with a range of intensity. When you add in the fact that you may feel a mix of two or more emotions at once, you may experience millions of feelings in the course of a single day. Welcome to the exhausting world of being human.

While we have some control over our feelings, you may find that what you wish you were feeling (gratitude, joy, triumph) is different from what you're actually feeling (boredom, fear, envy). The point of this chapter is that all feelings are valid feelings. Yes, every last one. And we don't want you to squelch any feelings or sweep them under the rug and pretend they're crumbs that you need to hide from visitors. We want to help you get comfortable with everything you're feeling by letting you know that you are completely normal.

Feelings aren't facts, but they *are* real and something happening inside your body and mind. Let's jump into exploring what you may be feeling now that you've found yourself unexpectedly in the role of caregiver.

Welcome to Caregiverland?

Chances are that you didn't expect to end up here. You likely made a vow during your wedding to care for each other in sickness and in health, or you may be a child who intellectually understood that the tables would one day turn and you'd be helping your parents instead of the other way around. But there is a big difference between knowing something may happen in the future and actually experiencing it in the here and now.

New caregivers are always battling with an element of surprise. Whether the aphasia is due to a sudden stroke or traumatic brain injury or comes on slowly due to a brain tumor or primary progressive aphasia, there is always a moment where you step over the line and find yourself suddenly in a new role: caregiver.

That new role brings with it thoughts and feelings. You may feel resentful because you had big plans for your own life or your lives together, and now you need to adjust those plans. You may feel grateful that the person is currently alive because it was touch-and-go for a while. You may feel helpless while you watch someone move from health to sickness. Or you may feel angry because no one can give you the concrete answers you crave.

It can be disorienting to find yourself in Caregiverland. No one aims for this place or particularly wants to stay here. But your stay will be a lot easier if you look around you. You are not the only person in Caregiverland. There are the people who work here, the people who live here—in other words, other caregivers, like you—and the people who have come to visit you. There is safety in numbers. In other words, don't try to navigate Caregiverland alone.

Mixed Emotions

Regardless of where you are in your caregiver journey, you are likely feeling a wide range of feelings. Guilt, resentment, frustration, hope, sadness, nostalgia, helplessness, and anger may crash over you in waves, sometimes tied to events and sometimes sneaking up on you without warning. You may be frustrated at your own confusion over the health care system while simultaneously being frustrated at your loved one for not practicing speech therapy exercises. You may be filled with happiness and hope while also filled with fear and dread—all at the same time.

All of this is normal, as well as the accompanying thoughts that stem from these feelings. You've lost control of the story of your life; this is not a chapter that you wanted to write. And unlike a job, this is not a position you can walk away from and feel okay leaving behind. You love the person in front of you, even if sometimes you don't like the person in front of you. Yes, even that is normal.

It's not the person you're frustrated with - it's the aphasia. And it's not even the aphasia - it's the lack of control. Aphasia spotlights a truth: we cannot control every situation and bend the world to our will. Confronting that fact day after day takes its toll.

You cannot hit rewind or call a do-over on life so things can go back to where they were before aphasia, but you can take steps to understand your emotions and feel as if you're walking alongside your feelings rather than being dragged through the day by them.

Chart Your Grief

Joe Biden (yes, as in the former U.S. Vice President) received advice for processing his grief after his wife's death and this exercise can help in any situation where a person is processing a life-altering situation. While Biden used it to chart grief, it can be used to chart any emotion.

This exercise came to Biden from the former governor of New Jersey. He told Biden what he began doing six months after his own wife's death, and how it helped him adjust to his new reality. In Biden's book *Promise Me, Dad*, he recounts the process on page 54,

> He told me to get a calendar, and every night, before I went to bed, put down a

number on that day's date. One is as bad as the day you heard the news, he said, and ten is the best day of your life. He told me not to expect any tens, and he said don't spend any time looking at that calendar, but mark it every day. After about six months, put it on graph paper and chart it. What he promised me turned out to be true: the down days were still just as bad, but they got farther and farther apart over time.

Charting gives you objective proof of your emotional journey rather than relying on the subjective nature of memory. You can look back at the months, seeing how you felt over time. That chart will hopefully change as you process your emotions.

This charting exercise works any time a person has a life-altering event where they need to come to a place of acceptance. You may still have down days, days where it is hard to accept the new normal, but those days will be farther apart once time passes. It's important to have visual cues to see how far you've come.

Emotions and Relationships

Aphasia changes relationships. The change may lean positive or negative, but you can't go through a major life upheaval and expect everything will continue on as is. Change isn't something to fear, but it *is* something to be realistic about.

Aphasia can test a relationship or marriage. Communication, a key piece of any relationship, whether with a spouse, parent, sibling, or friend, is suddenly inaccessible. Moreover, medical issues can change a person's personality or social skills. As a caregiver, you're going to need to weather these changes. Both sudden life-altering events and slow declines, such as primary progressive aphasia, affect how we interact with the world. People are forced to find unique ways to connect, including finding ways to minimize care-giver and care-receiver burnout.

For instance, if you're a caregiver for your spouse, you might try introducing a wordless date night into your weekly routine to have an escape from the speech therapy appointments and speech exercises.

Listen to music together. You don't need to leave the house to enjoy music. Settle in together and listen to a whole album from beginning to end. Of course, it's equally fun to go out and attend a concert. The newspaper often lists free performances in your area, or splurge and get tickets to your favorite show. And don't just head for the concert hall. You can find music in Irish pubs and jazz clubs. In fact, make it a game to try a different music venue every week.

Make your outings visual. Tour an art gallery, enjoying the paintings and sculptures. Become "photo tourists" and document an outing. You can use the camera on a phone or get a disposable camera at the drugstore. Look closely and take in the world around you. Give yourself a goal for the outing such as to photograph as many textures as possible or all objects of the same color. When you get home, look through the pictures you took together.

You don't need to go on a hike to get out in nature. Simply pick a beautiful spot — maybe a nearby park — and sit. You can engage in an activity, such as birdwatching, or simply enjoy the scenery and each other's company. Or take the wrong road. Look for roads that you've never turned down or intersections that you've passed through without wondering what is to the left or right. Taking a different turn sometimes means that you find interesting places close to home.

All of these ideas are equally applicable to any relationship: parent and child, friends, or siblings. Yes, relationships will change and that will bring with it a variety of feelings, but with work, you can steer some of those feelings towards happiness.

There Is Joy, Too!

Aphasia isn't just doom and gloom. It's not just problems and loss. Aphasia can bring two people closer together. In slowing life down, it can pare back the unimportant and leave behind newfound appreciation of the world around you. You will find new friends or new sources of strength. While no one wants aphasia in their life, there are silver linings when you find yourself confronting this communication disorder.

You can choose to accentuate the positive by celebrating small wins. Too often we wait to celebrate until we reach the endpoint, but what do you do when there is no endpoint? Or the endpoint is far off? With aphasia, the goal may be to return to the same communication ease that your loved one experienced prior to onset. And that is a great goal to strive for if you don't lose sight along the way that there will be plenty of smaller milestones that warrant attention and celebration, too.

Celebrations matter because they send a message to yourself and others: I've accomplished something and I'm proud. And you both should be proud! It is no small feat to have aphasia or be the caregiver for someone with aphasia. Celebrations send a message to the brain, giving it positive reinforcement. You may not have reached your end goal yet, but celebrating becomes an internal reminder that you've worked hard, and it makes you want to continue giving your all.

Celebrations are also about giving love to yourself or another person. It's a recognition of the value of effort, and it drives home a statement to yourself or to the person you're celebrating with: You matter, and I care about you. That is an important message to give yourself, too.

Celebrate the effort expended, especially the emotional energy invested in getting to this point. People are so much more than their aphasia, and celebrations acknowledge all other facets of a person's being.

Your celebration doesn't need to be a big party with a balloon release and confetti parade. Remember the list you made in Chapter 13 detailing the things that make you happy? Create a second list of things that make you *and* your loved one happy at the same time. They don't need to be grand gestures, but they should be actions that feel celebratory. Special meals, taking time for favorite activities, or spending time with someone you love can be ways of marking the moment.

The point isn't to just make this list, but to use it. If you do not have clearly defined goals you are attempting to reach, schedule your celebrations to mark ongoing actions. Maybe you want to celebrate attending speech therapy every four weeks or place a monthly "hard work celebration day" on the calendar so you remember to acknowledge work even if you haven't reached a specific milestone.

There is not a limit on how many celebrations a person can have; in fact, the more the merrier, since they become an ongoing reminder of the attempts made toward an end goal.

One Last Feeling

While we've covered many of the emotions you may be feeling, we barely scratched the surface of one of them: sadness. Caregivers get sad, too. Whether it is connected to your loved one's aphasia or due to everyday life, navigating sadness while you're focused on someone else can be a balancing act. In the next chapter, we'll specifically address dealing with sadness and getting help if your emotions become overwhelming.

CHAPTER 15: FINDING CARE FOR THE CAREGIVER

Your loved one with aphasia isn't the only person feeling sad and frustrated. Caregivers get sad, too. In fact, some get downright depressed. The Family Caregiver Alliance puts caregiver depression prevalence at a conservative 20% of all caregivers (which is double the rate of the general population), and the Mayo Clinic created a guide specifically for depression stemming from caregiving.

How can you best manage your sadness while helping a loved one through aphasia? This chapter specifically addresses sadness as well as solutions you may have been suspecting were going to be suggested to you all along: individual therapy and support groups.

What Causes Caregiver Depression?

Whether you call it sadness or depression, the fact remains that you're in an enormously stressful situation. Beyond fears of the unknown and the immense pressure on the caregiver to make continual decisions on another person's behalf, caregiving is exhausting. You're out of your routine and taking second place in your own life. You may not be eating well, exercising, or getting enough sleep. Your future has changed, and things you counted on may no longer be possible. If your daily communication partner is the person with aphasia, you may be missing your confidante. You may feel angry that things are progressing slowly, or frustrated with how long — and how many hoops you need to jump through — in order to get answers.

Caregiver sadness and depression is real and experiencing it doesn't mean that you're weak. It means that you're human and affected by the world around you. What counts is whether you treat it or dismiss it.

Turn to Your Support Circles

The first step in treating caregiver depression is prevention. Lean heavily on your circles of support and make sure you have adequate help so that all responsibilities don't fall squarely on your shoulders.

Your circle of support always has room to grow. There is the family we are born into and the "family" we create along the way. Being a caregiver opens you up to the possibility of bringing other caregivers into your fold. The other caregivers you meet at the hospital or speech therapy clinic form a like-experience support group of other people who "get" it.

Even if you have other people — friends and family members — to talk to, there is something special about sharing a difficult experience with someone who is going through the same thing at the same time. Just knowing you're not alone can go a long way in releasing some of the stress.

So strike up a conversation in the waiting room. That person sitting next to you may just become fictive kin. If you're not finding people to talk to, ask your doctor or speech therapist if they know other people in a similar situation that they can connect you with.

Release

If you don't have people to talk to, you might try releasing the stress by writing in a journal. Or open the voice memo app on your phone, go someplace quiet for a few minutes (the front seat of the car in the parking lot works), and just talk. Tell yourself how hard this is, how scared you are, and how frustrated you feel.

Writing it out in a journal has the added benefit of being a time capsule for those emotions. It can be empowering to look back on your words and know that you don't feel that same way anymore. It can also help you remember that you won't have your current feelings forever. Remember that chart you created in Chapter 14? Visuals are useful to return to when you're terrified a single feeling will last forever.

Also, our body has a natural way of releasing pressure: crying. Your body has this function for a reason, so take advantage of it! Let yourself have an all-out, puffy-eye crying session. Go somewhere private and let it out. Multitask and have a good cry in the shower so you can wash your face at the same time. Crying isn't a sign of weakness. Crying is a natural way to deal with stress and tension. Use it liberally to feel better.

Counseling and Support Groups

It can be invaluable to find a good counselor so you have a release valve for your feelings. Even if you only get to speak to your counselor occasionally, that time can improve your wellbeing, allowing you to express your fears and regroup. Counseling is important because you can say anything without feeling as if you're burdening a friend or family member with your feelings.

Counselors are trained to carry those heavy emotional loads. They aren't personally invested in the experience, so they have the distance to help you make sound decisions. There are counselors who use teletherapy, providing video counseling, which can be an option if getting to an office is not an option.

Think you don't have time for therapy? Similar to speech therapists, there are therapists who use teletherapy, providing a session via video or phone from the comfort of your own home. There are online therapy apps and websites, but some HMOs––such as Kaiser Permanente––offer remote therapy sessions under some plans. See if your insurance provider has the option for teletherapy or home-based therapy.

Many hospitals, rehab centers, and clinics offer support groups. Your loved one should join a support group with other people experiencing aphasia. It is valuable to connect with people who are going through a similar experience. There also might be a separate support group for caregivers. It's a chance to connect with other caregivers and share your highs and lows, all guided by someone knowledgeable about aphasia and/or caregiving.

The National Aphasia Association keeps an affiliate database so you can find services in your area. You can find clinics and support groups in your area by putting your ZIP Code into the database (https://www.aphasia.org/site/). But don't stop at our database. Conduct a Google search for "aphasia support group" + "your area" and see what comes up. If there isn't a support group, contact your speech therapy clinic or local hospital and suggest that they start an informal one. There is great comfort in spending time with other people who understand what you're going through.

Lining up Your Plan B

Caregiving is stressful, and because stress can lower your immune response, that stress sometimes causes physical illness in the caregiver. Therefore, caregivers always need to have a Plan B in place (remember Chapter 13) in case they need to step back due to illness.

That Plan B may include the number for a temporary home care agency that can connect you with an aide to get you through your illness, a neighbor or close friend who can step in at a moment's notice and help you out, or family members who can come visit and relieve you of your duties as you get well.

The No-Shame-Zone

Remember how we talked about the no-guilt-zone when it came to self-care? You also need to set up a no-shame-zone. There is no such thing as a bad emotion, and it is not a sign of weakness if you're feeling sad about your situation. Positive psychology is great, but we take things too far when we believe that we always need to stick to the sunny side of life.

When you encounter sadness, greet it like an old friend. Let it sit next to you, not on top of you. Acknowledge its presence as if it's an actual being in the room. Sadness has a way of making itself known, so if you ignore it, you're asking it to get your attention any way it sees fit.

We are almost at the end of our guide. We still have a few last words of advice to impart, though they're not actually from the NAA. They are from people with aphasia, professionals who work with aphasia, and other caregivers like you. It's powerful to learn from someone else's experience, and their words will let you know that you're on the right track as well as give you food for thought related to things you may want to try in the future.

Conclusion: Goodbye… and Hello!

We trust that you now know the lay of the land and you're feeling more confident as a caregiver. Feeling comfortable takes time, and some of it is tied to knowledge. The more you know, the more confident you'll feel, so set aside time each day to learn more about aphasia itself as well as the underlying cause of your loved one's aphasia, whether it is a stroke, traumatic brain injury, brain tumor, or primary progressive aphasia. The more you know, the better the caregiver you will be. You'll know the questions to ask, the therapies to explore, and the lingo to use to make your voice heard.

It may seem unbelievable today, but one day, your caregiving journey may come to an end or taper off as your loved one settles into their new normal and can do more things for themselves. In other cases, what is causing your loved one's aphasia may lead to the end of their life, and you will also move out of this caregiver stage of life. Like entering caregiving, leaving or changing the level of caregiving will bring with it big emotions, too.

Caregiver Layoffs

Provided your loved one doesn't push you away prematurely, every caregiver journey changes once your loved one can do things for themselves. They may still need your help for some tasks, but as much as you have longed to have the caregiving burden off your shoulders, it can be disconcerting when the day actually arrives.

It's a statement to how humans can get accustomed to anything, including aphasia stress. It's also a statement of how we can be happy and sad at the same time. You can be thrilled to have your time back while simultaneously sad that you're no longer deeply needed.

Except… you *are* needed. You're just needed in a different way. You still have a purpose, it's just a different purpose. So settle back into a new rhythm of companionship, enjoying the other person, and marveling at how far you've come together. Whether you're a child, parent, sibling, friend, or spouse, you have just gone on an intense journey together, and you will forever be connected through the hard work of coming through a crisis and finding new ways to communicate.

Caregiver Loss

But sometimes our caregiver journey comes to a different end. Primary progressive aphasia is a type of aphasia that doesn't have a cure and always moves to a resolution toward the end of life. Caregiver loss happens on two levels. There is the loss of your loved one that needs to be mourned, but there is also the loss of your role as a caregiver. It has been your role for a while, an identity that has been with you from morning to night. It's an adjustment to not only have your loved one gone but to have the rhythm of your day change once again due to that loss.

Unlike the caregivers above, you will not be able to marvel with your loved one of how far you have come together, but you will still have your circle of support to surround you in the aftermath. Let them know your needs, including whether you want a safe space to talk about your loved one and reflect on that caregiver journey. If your circle of support is small, please consider starting or continuing therapy. It is important not to carry the burden of loss on your own.

Your Thoughts

Of course, this is just the tip of the iceberg when it comes to advice. We are certain that there are great ideas that popped into mind—things you either do that would be helpful for other people to know or things that you wish you did (or, if you're a person with aphasia, that your caregiver did)—and we would love for you to share them so we can add them to the final version of this book.

If you have advice to pass along to other caregivers, please fill out our form. Just click that link, and it will open the form. We'll contact you if we're able to use it in the additional Chapter 16 that will appear in the final version of this book.

THANK YOU

Thank you for reading this guide. We hope that it was helpful. And we hope that you're hearing thank yous from your loved one, too. You are doing hard work as a caregiver that deserves to be acknowledged.

If you're not hearing enough thank yous, turn to this page and accept ours on behalf of the aphasia community: THANK YOU.

Thank you for being a caregiver. Thank you for stepping up and taking care of another person's needs. Thank you for the times you put yourself second so your loved one with aphasia can be first. We see you, we hear you, we're abiding with you, and we're always only a click away on the Internet, ready to provide information and support for both people with aphasia and their ever-important caregivers.

APPENDIX I

September 2020

	1 T
	2 W
	3 T
○	4 F
	5 S
	6 S
	7 M
	8 T
	9 W
	10 T
	11 F
	12 S
	13 S
○	14 M
	15 T
	16 W
	17 T
	18 F
	19 S
	20 S
	21 M
	22 T
	23 W
○	24 T
	25 F
	26 S
	27 S
	28 M
	29 T
	30 W

APPENDIX II

I HAVE APHASIA

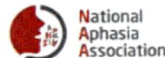

Aphasia is a communication disorder that affects a person's ability to understand, produce, or read written or spoken words. Aphasia presents differently in each person.

In fact, the only thing everyone with aphasia has in common is that aphasia does not affect the person's intellect.

Aphasia can occur after a head injury or stroke. It can also be the result of a brain tumor. In rare cases, aphasia is the result of primary progressive aphasia (PPA), which is a neurodegenerative disorder.

1. Communication Tips

Please keep your sentences short and simple. Give me time to think and respond. I can give you a thumbs up (yes) or thumbs down (no) sign in response to yes/no questions. Verify that we both understand what the other person is saying.

2. Please Contact

In case of an emergency, or if I'm unable to respond, please contact _____ at this phone number: _____.

3. Other Information

Change this section to add additional information specific to your loved one's situation or home.

Made in the USA
Monee, IL
03 December 2022